MOVE
AND HEAL

Feel Comfortable, Be Flexible

Move Well for Life in 3 Simple Steps

Edward Barrera

Disclaimer and Legal Notices

This Book is an educational health and fitness related information product.

The information presented within this Book solely and fully represents the view of the author as of the date of publication.

Understand that the information contained in this book is an opinion, and should be used for personal entertainment purposes only.

This book is not to be considered medical advice. Nor is this book to be understood as putting forth any cure for any type of acute or chronic health problems. The programs and information expressed within this book are not medical advice, but rather represent the author's opinions and are solely for informational and educational purposes.

The author is not responsible in any manner whatsoever for any injury or health condition that may occur through following the programs and opinions expressed herein.

Consult your doctor if you feel you need to.

Table Of Contents

Foreword

Within the sports science world, there are those rare moments when scientific research reveals a new twist on an old topic that gets your attention in a big way.

Pandiculation is one of those unique applications of neuroscience to change how we prepare to move well, compete and assists in the rehabilitation efforts of sports injuries and pain.

The old, traditional approach of stretch, stretch, stretch, is sadly behind the times in preparing our bodies for strenuous activities and in rehabilitating injuries and the discomforts that impede our life and competitive efforts. Since our muscles were designed to contract, isn't it logical that contractile applications will facilitate their true preparation for activity and bring them back into a state of normality when they have been injured or linger in discomfort.

The new frontiers of understanding brain plasticity have given us exciting insights into how basic motor activities can be controlled through brain-altering stimulation such as applied muscle contractions. Pandiculation takes these new revelations and effectively applies them to the sports, medical and integrative medicine worlds.

Edward Barrera is leading the way in his design of specific contractile muscle movements to prepare athletes and non-athletes for their sporting and physical pursuits. Pandiculation is the exciting application of the latest brain science that will benefit healthy and recuperating competitors and non-competitors alike on all levels.

- Timothy Berger, BA, MA, RN, ATC. Professor of Sports Science, Muskingum University

Author's Notes

Please enjoy my companion website where there is valuable information on moving comfortably for life.

You will also find links to my online digital products related to improving health and physical well being at GravityWerks.com.

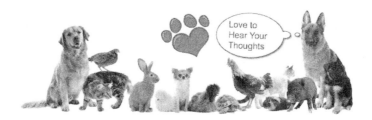

Thank you for purchasing my book. Please REVIEW this book. I need your feedback to make the next version better.

Thank you so much.

About the Author

Hi, I'm Edward Barrera, Hanna Somatic Educator® and founder of Gravity Werks. I teach people how to overcome physical pain, reduce muscular stress & tension, and recover quickly from injury with the little known animal act of pandiculation which, fortunately, has been systematized as somatics exercises, wherein we use a brain based approach of simple movement to quickly bring our body back to comfort, so we can get back out there and enjoy our physical pursuits.

This wasn't always the case for me, as I endured a near 2 decade long struggle of fibromyalgia/chronic pain during a career in the motion picture business where I worked as a Teamster, with the likes of Jeff Bridges, Kevin Costner, Tom Cruise, Chuck Norris, Oliver Stone and many others.

After trying scores of conventional and alternative health care methods, one fine day changed my life, when, for the first time, I felt surprisingly balanced and comfortable on account of certain postural correction exercises.

On this day, which took me 3 months in the program to get to, I wondered, if I could feel this way, how many others would no longer have to take the long road, like I did.

I learned a wonderful system known as Muscle Balance & Function Development® by Geoff Gluckman, similar to that used by Pete Egoscue®, where I was a client.

Along my merry way of getting back into sports, my knee meniscus tore and I literally stumbled my way into the world of somatics. *The body experienced from within*, as defined by Thomas Hanna, the author of *Somatics* and the creator of Hanna Somatic Education.

During the 3 year training to become a Hanna Somatic Educator, in which we learned to be both bodyworker and movement coach, my world view turned upside down about my understanding of exercise and stretching.

Mel Siff, author of *Facts and Fallacies of Fitness*, said, programming the central nervous system (the brain) is the most important aspect of all exercise—far more important than strength training or aerobics. It must never be neglected.

What I came away with is the approach all healthy animals with a spine on the planet use to remain flexible, mobile, comfortable and pain free in order to maintain the agility required to *Move Like an Animal.*

It's my hope and desire to bring you back to what you already intuitively know and have most likely have forgotten to do if you continue to live in pain or discomfort or can't recover like you used to. *Our birthright is to move well* at all stages in our life. The natural act of pandiculation is a profoundly simple act using the brain's cortex to reprogram our movement software. This is the very one in which our fellow healthy animals show us how to remain free from stiffness, retain our agility and keep our mobility and flexibility intact.

With greater freedom in our bodies, our minds expand with the possibilities of truly moving well as we age. We can comfortably manage and self-correct as nature intended.

For those of you who have tried a lot of approaches or are ready to cross the rubicon, see the matrix, or go down the rabbit hole and want to dig deeper into the mind-body connection, the simplicity of pandiculation is a profound paradigm shifter.

... and it's best said by the people I've had the great pleasure to impart this too.

"It's so too simple".

"This boggles the mind but not the body".

"I'm already starting to feel the positive effects of this method. It's crazy, but the smaller I make my movements, the more relief it seems to bring. It makes no sense, but I don't care!"

The human animal can tap back into our very own natural self-corrective central nervous system programming ways so we can unleash the power of the brain to be comfortable, flexible and move well for life.

It's been a source of great pleasure to have lived pain free these past 16 years, win medals at the state and national levels and help many people rediscover the fountain of youth. Pain and discomfort can be one of our greatest teachers and we can learn to master its signal to move well for life or simply to *Move Like an Animal*.

Edward

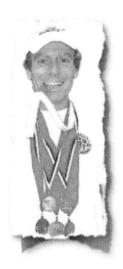

Thanks

Thanks to my wonderful editors, Rebecca Simpson, MA, and my dear Laurie Sterling whose kind patience and wonderful heart is a blessing.

A special thank you to our fantastic exercise photographer, Natasha Sterling. Go Tasha!

And to you Mom and Dad. Thanks for all your love and support.

Introduction

Are you still stiff when you wakeup and it's hard to get out of bed?

Does your body no longer recover like it used to?

Does the pain, ache, stress and tension continue even if you do nothing?

Have you tried everything with no lasting relief?

To be able to move comfortably, easily and freely as you once did may seem like a forgotten memory or ability. It's our **birthright to move well** and keep it that way as we age.

Wonder how healthy animals remain limber, agile, flexible, are balanced and retain vitality? After all, when is the last time you saw a cheetah run 60 mph and pull a hamstring? All it takes for us is to reach, bend or roll over in bed and ouch! go our muscles as we end up with a painful spasm or cramp.

Our brain has the very software we can simply use to update ourself back to comfortable levels. And no you won't need a teenager to reprogram your own movement system back online. See, this is what babies and healthy vertebrate animals use on daily basis to move with ease.

Even if we've gotten a little off track, like I did in my 20's & 30's. I endured the misery of chronic pain and earned the diagnosis of fibromyalgia. That's chronic body wide pain and "they" called it incurable. Now 16 pain free and comfortable years later, I learned and remembered how to *Move Like an Animal*.

Now I can ROAR and feel good everyday, while teaching thousands of people how to regain mobility, restore natural flexibility, reduce stress and tension, and recover quickly from injury using a specific part of the brain where we can self-adjust our own muscular and movement system levels back to comfort. This is so easy and anyone can do it.

Getting older can be full of graceful, free flowing movement where all the stress rolls off us like a duck rolling its feathers.

You can return to physical activity where no soreness, stiffness, aches and the need for a hot tub or ice disappears.

Lori couldn't drive a car anymore in comfort and she would be brought to tears with the pain. Now she can drive comfortably and loves to free up her muscles as easily as any healthy animal does. Driving a car is now a piece of cake for this busy Mom.

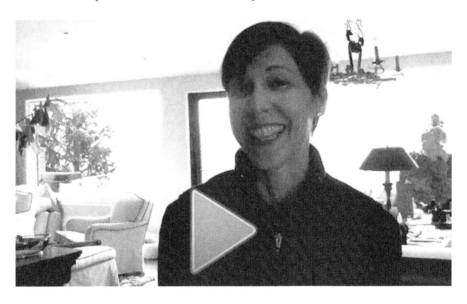

Watch: http://www.youtube.com/watch?v=XvOeGF4bJ4Y&feature = c4-overview&list=UU1zyMpVarOtM040yNtD0z3g

When David got his back spasms in his 40's from painting underneath a boat. The twisting motion laid him out and he lived with a back which would go out and he'd have to deal with back spasms. At 72, he learned how to move like an animal again - and no more back spasms.

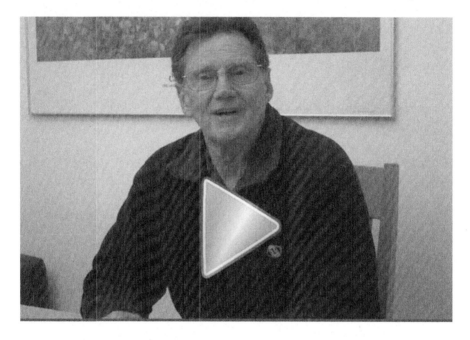

Watch: http://www.youtube.com/watch?v=0PP8Jn8eX1o&list=UU1z yMpVarOtM040yNtD0z3g

When Debbie, a nurse, had a heavy man fall on her and cause her to have chest pains. Her doctor gave her some pills. When she got home, still in pain, she remembered to do the movements she was taught and the pain was gone. No need for those pills after all.

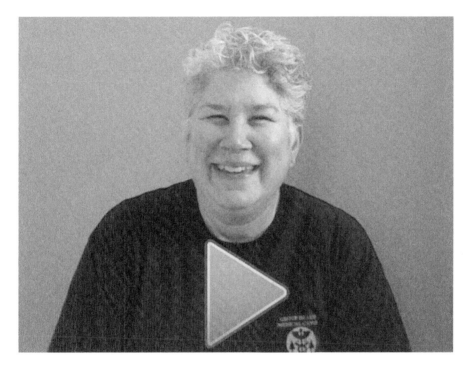

Watch: http://www.youtube.com/watch?v=is1dAhIn1Ng&list=UU1z yMpVarOtM040yNtD0z3g

Mary Lou was slated for back surgery and attended a workshop where she learned how to move like an animal. Afterwards she went on vacation. When she returned, she cancelled the surgery.

Here's what they're saying:

Hi Ed. I am another of your success stories--I was on a plane to Alaska, and a 12 day whirlwind trip around Anchorage and the Kenai Penninsula by car. I was pain free and full of energy--while I kept doing my 3 favorite back movements!

I called the neurosurgeon and canceled a scheduled back surgery on my return home! At my last two chiropractic appointments, no adjustment was needed!

- Marilu, WA

Now how long do you want to continue hanging onto that old friend of pain, stiffness, immobility or the inability to let tension finally go. When you finish reading this book, you'll know how to *Move Like an Animal* and the 3 steps it takes to let go of all the pain, stiffness, discomfort, tension, stress and even possibly save you from surgery.

Turn the page and you'll remember how to M*ove Like an Animal*; feel comfortable, be flexible, and move well for life in minutes.

Chapter 1

What is the Animal Secret to Moving Well and Being Comfortable for Life? Even Babies Know How to Do It...

Wouldn't you agree that animals move incredibly well? Do you marvel at their agility, flexibility, balance and poise? Do you ever see them going to their secret gym where they become adept at moving well? How have they hidden from us their secret moves which allow them the agility and flexibility to swoop, jump, twist and turn effortlessly?

How do you feel when your muscles let go of the stress and tension you take on every day? How long has it been? Isn't it wonderful when the feeling of relaxation flows through your muscles as if you've come out of a hot tub or a "good hands" massage?

Isn't that sleepy, yawning, relaxed feeling so exquisite that you wish it came in a bottle? Go ahead—take a sip and re-lax. That's right, let go. Easier said than done...

Babies and animals know how to create relaxation and move well while many adults remain in the mystery and in misery with the aches and pains of getting older and stiffer.

The Secret Training Gym

Fido and the very young know where the "secret training" gym is to move well for life. Every day they show us what to do to remain in good health with, arguably, the world's largest exercise system on the planet which most doctors and physical educators aren't even aware of.

1

Back in 1680, the founder of modern clinical medicine, Herman Boerhaave, noted that a certain act would bring muscles to rest.

Ironically, he and many others up until the present day have been studying yawning. Now there's a subject to get relaxed over.

The "P" Word

What he noted may seem to be a rather strange sounding word. When is the last time you *pandiculated* in public?

You see, a pandiculation is a 3 part act in which we contract certain muscles in act 1. Take a yawn for instance. Go ahead, give it a shot.

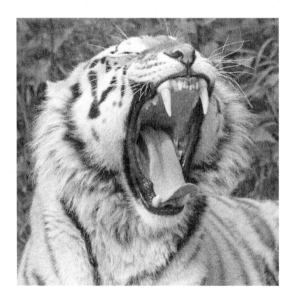

Open wide and feel which muscles you are using. Certainly, you can feel your jaw tighten. Can you feel how the front of your neck is contracting? If you open your mouth a little and pull the jaw back and talk, you can feel how your voice changes as you keep what is called the platsyma held in a state of tension.

Now try again and open the mouth wide and notice if you feel your shoulders moving back. Try once again and find out if you feel your hips moving ever so slightly.

You may not notice the subtle shift, which is OK. If you did feel it, you may already be starting to become relaxed by all the conscious yawning.

Welcome to the world of the healthy animal and youthful movement practice.

To Stretch or Not to Stretch?

So here's a question. What is the first thing your pet cat or dog does in the morning? Before they check their email and make a cup of coffee, what is it that they do?

They stretch. Right? Wrong!!!

Animals with a spine are not stretching. I know you're thinking, *Well yes, Ed, they are*. Are you so sure? Whenever a cat rounds its back what we see appears to be a stretch.

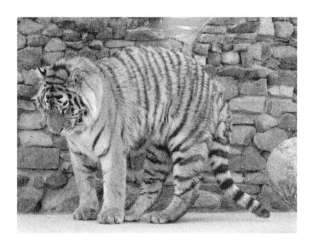

This is not what the big cat is actually doing, even though it appears as if it is right before our eyes, so bear with me for a moment.

Instead, she is contracting her belly, pulling it in and using those muscles so it appears as if she is stretching or rounding the back.

Go for it; pull your belly in as if you are rounding your back and feel how the belly tightens, the chest sinks down and even the pubic bone lifts up—that is, if you still have that type of mobility which, by the way, you can recapture at any age.

This is what vertebrate animals do to set themselves up for successful movement, whether it's a frog, dog or elephant in the room. Before they go out, you'll see them contract in various ways or maneuvers. They'll do about 7 to 10 of these things first thing in the morning. And here we were, thinking they were just being cute all along.

Right under our noses they've been showing us what to do. Not stretch, rather contract muscles which have naturally shortened overnight.

Don't you feel a little stiffer when you wake up? If you're a healthy vertebrate animal then you too would normally reach an arm or arms, extend the legs, arch your back and other apparently seeming stretching maneuvers. All along, your brain has been getting the message to contract muscles along a certain chain which is part of your movement system.

When you get to that morning stretch the next time, pay attention to what it is you are contracting. You see, muscles are designed to do one thing only. They receive a message from the brain to contract. We'll cover more of how we can use the brain and body in the next chapter.

What is the Animal Secret to Moving Well and Being Comfortable for Life? Even Babies Know How to Do It...

The Act of Pandiculation

This formerly known act of a stretch forms the first part of a pandiculation. When you watch Fido let go, you might see him hesitate a little as a limb returns. There may be a little shimmy or jerky type of quality as he moves back towards where he started. Of course, you won't see him holding any pose for any length of time or counting 1-2-3 6 seconds let go, reach a little further. No, instead, he does a simple contraction along a series or chain of muscles and then a letting go. That is part 2 of the 3rd act of a pandiculation.

Throughout the course of a day and even before bedtime, another set of pandiculations will occur so that some 40 - 50 of these mindful contraction movement patterns will have taken place.

How to Be Limber and Agile

This is what sets them up for successful movement and keeps them limber and agile throughout the course of a day and lifetime. Even after they've been freaked out—which you'll see when they shake themselves about—they let the accumulated stress roll off of them like a duck ruffling its feathers.

Now what about those babies in the mother's womb? Just ask Mom if she felt you moving around, apparently not stretching your limbs, instead contracting your fetal muscles as you learned how to develop your initial movement and built your foundation for successful movement.

Movement System Update Software

Naturally, you had the good sense to practice this out of the womb until sometime later in life when many of us literally forgot how to reset and update our movement system, much in the same way as we update our computers.

We all know our computers have to keep up with updates; otherwise they become outdated and slow. Hmm, sound familiar?

In the next chapter, we'll delve a little deeper into how the brain is highly involved in the healthy animal secret to moving well and keeping us comfortable for life.

Turn the page now to find out how the brain can reset muscles to regain comfort and how we can turn off stiffness, immobility and pain...

Chapter 2

How do You Get Less Stiff, Feel More Flexible and Get Rid of Pain?

Now that you understand how animals set themselves up for successful movement, how can we use the «p» word to transform the root cause of our stiffness and physical pains?

Wouldn't you like to be able to zap painful, discomforting signals sooner rather than later?

Muscles are subject to commands from the brain. When you point your finger at someone, or some object, there is a set programmed length for you to reach your arm. This programming is what we rely on to drive and text if you're a teenager. The rest of us may be too stiff to multi-task and rather not take certain risks. Sometimes, stiffness is a good thing.

Learned Movement

The sub-cortical areas of the brain are the places where our learned programs reside. This is so we can move without thinking about every step.

When we adapt and learn something new, we shift into another part of our brain, the cortex.

The Feedback Loop

In terms of movement and feelings or sensations, we have a motor-sensory cortex which forms a feedback loop of information which flows in the spine. As we intend to move, information flows back up for us to sense and feel our way with it.

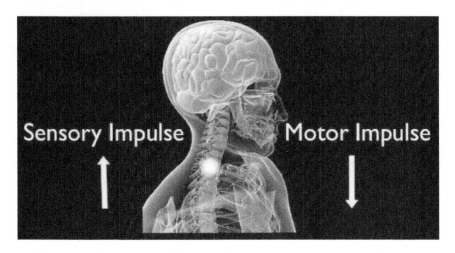

When we consciously think about moving a certain part of ourself, we rev up the motor in the brain's cortex. We can use this part of the brain to pay attention to how our motor operates.

The sensing part of the brain gets to feel the self-adjustments and the quality of the feel of our movements.

The Highway of Information

The information highway, or nervous system, gets well programmed so most our movements are done without any particular awareness on our part. Once learned, we move on.

When we think of the nervous system revving itself up, we're in what is called the sympathetic state. When we turn things down and return to states of calmness and relaxation; we're in our parasympathetic state.

When we live with increasing tension, high stress levels, we tend to feel and process this flow of information as if our motor is «on» and we can't seem to idle down or allow the muscles or tension to fully rest or relax.

Is Letting Go Easy?

Just let go ... easier said than done if your nervous system is on high alert. If you «try» to find the «off» switch or button, it may not get turned off or you may no longer remember how to access it.

Even at rest, the brain's sub-cortical areas will keep the on-going program vigilantly ready to go or bracing the muscles to states of being bound up.

Naturally, we think we oughta be able to sleep and wake up rested and comfortable. Yet, at night, muscles tend to shorten.

What Does the Healthy Animal Do?

The animal thing to do, of course, is to wake up the nervous system by pandiculating out the tightness and stiffness which naturally occurs.

Fido, as you learned in the first chapter, has this down. Fido goes cortical and begins the day by setting himself up for successful movement. That'll keep one's tail wagging.

Are You in the Loop?

The brain's cortex is designed to release tension levels when we use the feedback loop of the motor-sensory system along with another loop called the alpha-gamma loop.

Neurons, which are cell bodies, extend and communicate. Our

body is communicating at various levels throughout our entire existence. We've learned, through neural plasticity, that the brain can change so the muscles which receive information from the brain can also change and be updated, much like a computer which needs software updates to help it run more smoothly and effectively.

The alpha system contracts to create the necessary tension to move our bag of bones around.

The gamma system gives you the sense of movement.

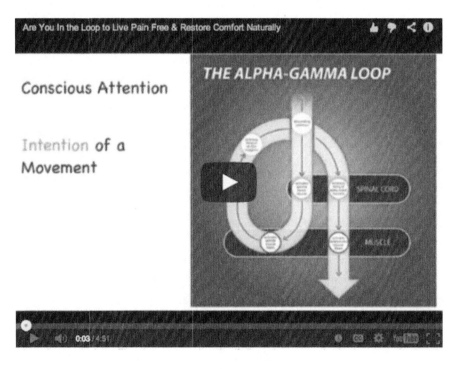

Watch the video at http://youtu.be/R4A8OjeOfQo for a fuller explanation.

This loop is what we can manage and change to alter how well we move and how we feel our movement taking place.

Overcoming Feelings of Pain - The Reset Button

In the pain management field, we've come to see how people can successfully overcome physical pain, stiffness, stress and high tension levels since the cortex is set up to release tension.

In the same way a thermostat regulates itself, we can bring our comfort levels to where we want them by using the brain and our intention to move. We simply reset and move on.

When we consciously focus our intention—and pay attention to how the brain organizes our "letting go" of a movement pattern—we're more aware of the 2 parts of our animal pandiculation action.

The performing of a movement is one thing. Its undoing entertains us with possibilities you'll learn about in chapter 4.

This reset button we touch primes the brain to release chemicals of relaxation more powerful than a hot tub. It un-locks the stiff «holding» information and resets the brain's sub-cortical programs. Now we can drive, text and reach for the bag of cookies in the back seat without harming ourselves or others.

Stretch Reflex 101

When we've experienced tight, stiff muscles, many of us have been taught to stretch it out, not realizing the nature of how the brain's programming system works.

Mabel Todd noted, in the 1930's, that when the athletes she worked with stretched a contracted muscle, the muscles would re-contract and re-tighten.

When we place our hands near a hot stove, we reflexively pull back. This lightning fast reflex happens when we pull a muscle or get a calf cramp or back spasm. Ouch!

What most likely happens is that our muscles are already tensing at higher levels in the first place. We move in a certain way and ouch! go the lights as the message doesn't have to reach the brain, it'll happen quickly from the spinal cord.

Protection Mode

Now we're in protection mode and the slightest of movements can cause that sudden twinge or twang of pain. Now we're locked with nowhere to go, hoping it goes away as suddenly as it came on.

Sometimes we stay stuck-on since the brain is not being re-programmed to let go of the holding tension.

How to Unlock Tension, Stiffness and Pain; Let's Go Cortical

Un-locking and un-binding our tight and over-contracting tensed muscles is easy once you know or remember how to do it.

In the same manner as homeopathy works, we use the signal the brain is sending rather than pulling against it to reinforce the tension level. Instead, when we go cortical by consciously increasing the rate of contraction, as we decrease this with our conscious attention, our muscles do the most extraordinary thing—they remember to let go.

In this sense, the body knows where neutral is, otherwise we couldn't shift to our parasympathetic, more relaxed states.

When we use the brain's cortex, the pump of relaxation flows. We rebuild our reservoir so we can have our stress and eat it too. Yummy!

Letting go of high tension and tight, stiff muscles isn't easy if you're accustomed to the brain's program holding you in check or restricting movement you've adapted to for a number of reasons, we'll talk about it in the next chapter.

By «going cortical», you get back in control and take out the very «charge» of the feelings of restriction, renewal resurfaces and the muscles feel comfy once again.

Recap

Healthy animals pandiculate. When we do the same and pay attention to our movement, we go cortical and we can notice how the brain organizes the muscles as we release. Relaxation returns.

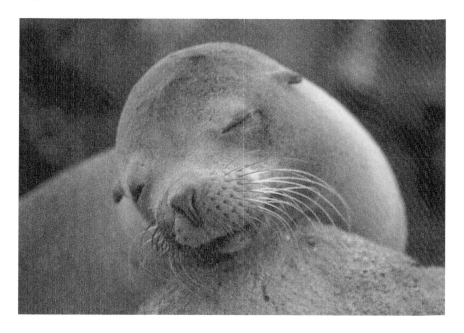

The upside is that the muscles regain lost function as the holding pattern diminishes.

The two parts of a pandiculation now set us up for the entire 3 part act you'll learn to do for yourself in chapter 4. Before we go there, we'll take a look at what gets in our way. Turn the page to see how we can reverse engineer compensations and pain to move well for life.

Chapter 3

What do Compensations have to do with Pain and Discomfort?

To move like a comfortable animal, we have to look to our ability to be as functional and aware of our body as possible, given our present circumstances.

Our past history of falls, sprains, strains, accidents, traumatic events, injuries, family modeling, peer togetherness, accumulation of stress, sports and physical activity cueing can have a detrimental effect and lead us to compensation patterns.

Do you want to move comfortably for the rest of your life?

Do you want to know what it is that prevents you from moving well and interfering with your physical activities?

Do you think it is possible to change your body and that you have the power to do so?

Well let's go on with your bad%#s animal self. ROAR!

You can R-O-A-R back and recover-over-any-restriction which gets in the way by routinely pandiculating.

You can un-do movement habits and compensation patterns and recover from current or past injuries. You can give up the hobbling, stiff or bound up movements when you understand how compensations can bring us down.

What Are Compensations?

The ideal or neutral alignment posture is when our ankles are underneath our knees. Our knees are underneath our hips. The hips lie underneath the shoulders in a more vertical line.

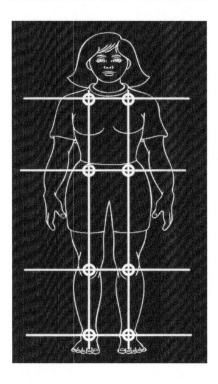

Ideally, we see this alignment both in the front and back side of ourselves. From both of our sides, again the ideal relaxed posture is in line and our head is ideally centered.

There is no bracing or holding one's self up. When we have equal tension, we stand comfortably in the ever present field of gravity.

Another measure is to look at horizontal levels of the shoulders, hips, knees and ankles.

Since we're all unique in terms of our size, length of our bones, and weight, things may not appear as uniform. When we take a deeper look, ideal function can happen when our joint centers mentioned above are more in alignment rather than the tissue or skin levels we think we see.

We can twist, swing, bend and reach more easily when things are more coordinated with movement being displaced from our center of gravity.

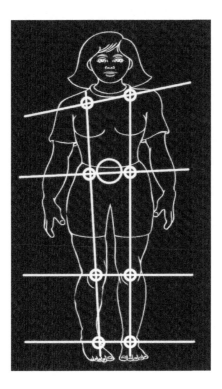

When our center of gravity is being displaced on a day to day basis, as it is with compensations, we'll move as best as we can given our present circumstances.

When one of these vertical or horizontal lines is out of whack—one being higher or lower than another, more forwards or shifted backwards or showing a rotation—a combination of an elevation, shift forwards, and rotation can also take place as a multi-dimensional compensation. Now that's holding it in place.

Can Compensations Shift?

There was a time when we believed compensations are fixed. You might have figured you have some type of structural quirk you have to live with. Maybe you thought *this is the way I'm built and this is how my body does things*.

Today, we can see postures shift before our eyes. People are reporting that the pain, stiffness, or discomfort feels better.

The question I had, as a former chronic pain sufferer, was, *but will it hold? Will this new posture which can feel very different, or renewed set of comfortable feelings, last?*

Movement itself is a set of learned actions. We all had to build ourselves up step by wobbly step in order to balance and then walk in victory.

In the course of life, we can take our share of falls, sprains, and strains. No big woof, or so we think. We collect trauma, hobble around and use other muscles to do the normal job of getting us around.

How Do Compensations Continue?

Then we might go into protection mode and use other muscles in order not to flinch with more discomfort. I know I used to stop going there when it hurt only to be painfully reminded when I forgot not to go there.

This type of remembering can keep the splint, bracing, favoring one leg and protection meter on until we figure out another way to shift or we heal enough and feel ready to go again.

So naturally we substitute other muscles and movement arrangement patterns until we begin to adapt and move around the best we can.

In the long run, any number of injuries and the onslaught of stresses we face can take its toll and our body can withdraw into it's self, while we keep trying to hold it all together. Whew, sounds like a lotta hard work and energy. No wonder I felt tired and wiped out even after a night's sleep.

Then there are the everyday things we do, such as carrying a purse or backpack primarily on one side and keeping that shoulder higher. In time, the muscles do this «go to» program.

Holding your telephone with your ear to your shoulder can create a holding compensation, maybe this is why some of us love the speakerphone when the shoulder or neck begins to ache. Of course, now you may be keeping the arm bent and the bicep muscle stays contracted as we adapt to keeping our arm more bent over time with our smart phones.

The clothes we wear can restrict certain movements. Even those high heels will keep the calf muscles looking nice and tight—until they feel rock hard and you no longer remember to let go. There's gotta be some kid out there thinking about a hydraulic set of high heels so you can low ride when your legs are back under the desk or table.

Since we're all a bunch of animals built with a monkey-see monkey-do capacity, we may think of movement as a genetic pattern inherited from our family to move in a certain way. We simply learn by those around us; we can model our speech and movement habits. Since

I "growed" up in Texus, ya'll know what I'm talkin 'bout. Thus I learned my former cowboy bow-legged walk wasn't going to serve me in the long run.

Today, when we look around, we see a number of duck walkers with feet and knees splayed out.

The gamers and book worms as we called them, can end up with rounded or curved spines from spending a lot of time enjoying themselves.

Our everyday innocent activities can lead us down the path of compensations which build up over time. We're programming our muscles to certain go-to patterns.

Sitting Kills

Then there is the silent killer of sitting. Remember when Mom or Dad laid into us to sit up straight? OK, how many of you felt the urge to sit up now? When that program is a «go» a little hint or reminder will do.

Certain cueing may have over activated us to respond or brace—if we'd rather slump in defiance or we are truly beat from sitting at our desks and taking on all the stress work brings. Our body will be used in a way to follow our habit or tension we can't let go.

Today, our sedentary lifestyle of eating at a table, working at a desk, sitting to watch entertainment, driving a car, all leads up to a whole lotta sitting, folks. Even people who exercise cannot negate the effects of all the sitting we've accustomed ourselves to. I mean, what would happen if they gave the school bus drivers a day off and didn't allow the parents to drive the kids to school? Oh the horror!

While paying attention to our posture is all well and good, it's possible we've lost certain functions or connections to how well we feel when our posture is aligned. It actually feels better to sit upright when tension patterns are more balanced. At the same, it is perfectly normal to let it all hang down when things need to. The trap is when this normal hangs on for too long or we keep playing the unconscious habit.

Our animal friends, predators and the hunted alike can still favorably lounge, sit and move about unless they compensate which brings them to a swifter end.

We can keep on going. But at what cost for how long?

Will the proprioceptive police show up at your door? Can you be arrested for being a proprioceptive illiterate?

One of my mentors, Thomas Hanna, who created Hanna Somatic Education and developed somatics exercises, said we folks here in the good ol' US of A... "are a nation of proprioceptive illiterates".

When we are able to sense our alignment, not by seeing if things are aligned yet, but by feeling our sense perceptions as we use our body in our various activities, we can adjust ourselves back to comfort.

The pain, discomfort, tightness and stiffness come after being out of longer term alignment while keeping the stress on the tissues or having stress further wear us down.

When I'm a bit cranky or out of sorts, people seem to scatter or want to battle. The proprioceptive police are right around the corner reminding me I could self-adjust before things get too far gone.

The signs of groaning to get up out of a chair, that spasm which keeps us up at night, the inability to recover like you used to, the niggling tension or stress which isn't resolving are indicators the proprioceptive police are headed to your door. The good news is, you're already arrested and we save tax dollars by not having Congress create this separate police force even though their now former separate healthcare system can't keep this police from showing up at their door too.

But hey, don't get me going on the postures of our elected leaders.

Can Having a Compensation Make Exercise or Recovery Difficult?

When you're going into your gym, exercise program, doing yoga or physical activity such as gardening and you're already compensating, you'll move in the best way you can.

The flip side is you're most likely reinforcing compensations with a particular exercise or repetitive movement which adds to the physical issue.

Many athletes, at least the weekend and weekday warriors I play with, along with the people in the gym, are still in pain. I see them take their ibuprofens, stretch lamely for a few seconds, wear the same braces year after year and keep hearing the mantra of "I have to get in shape".

I don't think it's a matter of getting in shape. That is always an evolving concern. The key is to be able to recover and move comfortably and not hobble your way back to the car or cart in between holes, sets or games.

Exercise in many forms oughta be more beneficial than the less optimal ways I see people going at it. If your body isn't recovering like it used to... Houston, we gotta problem.

Running Out of Energy

As we move around in a compensated body, we're more likely to expend more energy than necessary. Instead of idling at neutral, we're already revved up and then we can't downshift later on. Then, when we go in for a pit stop, it's "Where's the hot tub, ibuprofen, tiger balm, ice or red wine?"

We're working a little harder and breaking down more quickly so the pains, stiffness and braces remain until we take self-corrective action.

A secret tip: After a soccer game I'll hear I was all over the place in terms of running. Maybe yes, but not so much. What's going on is this: People's compensation patterns are running them out of gas, then when I putter by them it looks like I've gained speed. It's a matter of timing and waiting for the inevitable breakdown to occur. I'd rather finish strongly and be able to play again then wear myself out completely simply on account of function failing too early.

When I see a fellow aligned athlete who is compensating less, then there's some competitive work and fun to be had.

Regaining function and relaxing muscles back into neutral alignment allows the restoration of the muscles which can provide us with ample energy. The renewal happens quite readily as the brain is set up for it, if we only dare tap into it.

How Do We Reverse Engineer a Compensation and Un-compensate and Get Out Of Pain More Quickly?

Getting muscles to return to function and to coordinate movement actions or patterns is how animals naturally set themselves up, as we discussed in chapter 1. In other words, mindful pandiculations help us reset our body back to comfort.

Moving in more connected ways repairs us so we can go on more confidently and we swim in our own inner hot tub as our brain can create incredible relaxation by adjusting tension levels through the act of a pandiculation, as we learned in chapter 2.

When we reset our own tension levels, the muscles feel softer and more comfortable. Those bones which are being pulled into a certain position can now shift out of a held compensation program. The very pain we were sensing or feeling begins to soften away.

Instead of fighting pain, we "go with it" to dissolve it.

The very release of our muscle tension then shifts the bones instead of rebalancing muscles as we attempt to do in regular exercise. We re-regulate and self-adjust tension as we remember to move like an animal. Go ahead—purr, slink and melt the tension so the jaw is slack again.

In regular exercise, we attempt to go for balance and strengthen weakness. All well and good; you can achieve an upright posture, good alignment and feel good. I taught a wonderful system known as Muscle Balance and Function Development, by Geoff Gluckman, where we rebalanced a person by doing the opposite of what they were doing. We looked at the compensation patterns and how people are out of certain planes and ranges of movement. Then we systematically applied exercises to restore the planes back to neutral and help rebalance muscles and people felt better. It's a great system and similar to Pete Egoscue's method which is more muscularly based than the plane method.

It wasn't until I had a knee meniscus torn that I learned about another system called somatics exercises which were seemingly easy, simple movement patterns founded on the pandicular process. I was able to rehab quite quickly and move far better than before. That got my attention.

Going Down the Rabbit Hole

I had been "doing" exercise and now my muscles and movement system felt much softer, less contracted, less tense and it was far easier to move. I began to feel the tai chi movements I had been practicing in a completely different manner.

Sometimes a paradigm shift can feel a little odd yet, intuitively, our body has such great wisdom. My concept of exercise began to shift as I gave up traditional stretching, later on learning how much of it is no longer supported or at least there is a great debate going on. Many trainers have completely abandoned it and are trying other methods.

As a newfound sense of mobility and a restoration of natural flexibility returned, I was able to move comfortably and the knee was no longer an issue and, surprisingly, ever since then I've continued to increase my function by not training like I used to.

Now, I merely move like an animal and I recover, renew and restore the muscles and movement system. Naturally, this is happening for the thousands of people I've worked with and who have learned the simple 3 step method of somatics exercises you're going to learn how to do for yourself.

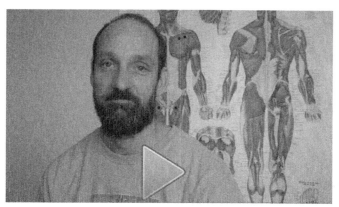

Watch the video at http://youtu.be/rsIJe--QbRo. Hear how Sean can do sports and not have any pain or stiffness anymore.

Recap

The compensations we once thought of as fixed can be shifted. The results are feelings of well-being and more energy. Through a natural, simple resetting of tension levels we move like an animal again, a more comfortable one which rebuilds function and renewal simultaneously.

Now that you know about compensations and animal pandiculations and you've been introduced to somatics exercises, let's put all of this together.

In the next chapter, you'll learn the 3 step method to regain mobility, restore natural flexibility, reclaim vitality and feel comfortable to move well for life.

Turn the page now to learn the 3 step method.

Chapter 4

What is the 3 Step Method to Feel Comfortable, be Flexible and Move Well for Life?

When a cat wakes up in the morning, she'll do her usual 7 - 10 pandiculation maneuvers in the morning to reset tension levels. Remember, she's not stretching.

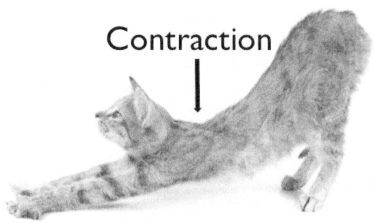

Contraction = Pandiculation

If we continue our stretching ways, we may violate the stretch reflex switch you learned about in chapter 2.

Naturally, she has reset her muscles for another vital day of movement. These types of waking up movements make up the heart of the 3 step method used in somatics exercises.

Even a duck contracts a number of muscles along a certain coordination chain. When the duck releases the now shortened muscles, often you'll see a little hesitation or jerky quality as the brain's motor cortex regains control.

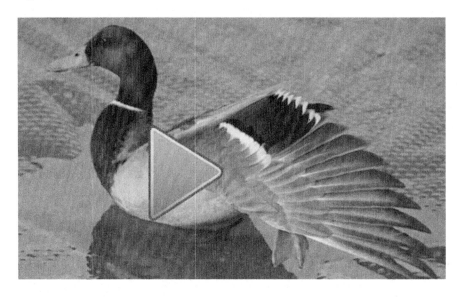

Watch the video at http://youtu.be/FLEr-Dd1xjY to see how you too can ruffle your feathers so tension and stress leaves your body.

You won't see an animal hold a so-called stretch for any length of time. The happy pandiculator moves to a destination and then reverses course. There is a measured contraction or shortening of muscles followed by a release back to where things started.

The muscular reset phase happens as the brain dumps relaxation chemicals. Now those muscles are relaxed and ready for action. Would you like to be able to have your brain turn on the free drugs spigot?

For the human animal, the actions work about the same, except that a majority of us have forgotten to do this over time. We've become compensated; we've adopted poor posture and poor movement habits which have served us a plate full of the stiffness, immobility, aches and the strains we live with.

To remember how to do this may take some getting used to though, intuitively, when you release the relaxation chemicals, you're back home in the comfort zone. Then the reset happens very quickly.

Since we did this as babies and young children, we're just going to have to deal with our larger bones, weightier self and the compensations we can unwind in time.

The Reverse to Most Approaches

Unlike regular exercise or the striving for more range of motion, this is more about quality than quantity. This approach is the reverse of most approaches out there. I often call this un-exercise, since you're attempting to un-do tightness and un-lock stiffness so comfort readily returns.

This is done gently and with less effort than regular exercise.

You're rebuilding the foundation for movement itself.

WARNING

If you push your muscles, the good news is you did it. Yeah! If you do it too fast or with too much effort, what can happen is that you may push the stretch reflex mechanism into the "on" position. The muscles will tighten back up to their previous set program or a muscle spasm may turn on.

Releasing set tension levels is best afforded with gentle, easy, mindful movement.

What is the 3 Step Method and How Can You Use it?

The simple 3 steps are "oh so too simple" as a client told me. This may "boggle the mind but not the body".

Most of us are used to the striving, pushing or going for range of motion type of movements where we exert ourselves to go a little more, a little further. This is the complete reverse since you're working with your brain's motor cortex which works when you move with the least amount of effort.

By paying attention during the entire movement sequence, your brain will handle the details. All we gotta do is stick to the 3 part act as closely as possible.

Here are the 3 Steps

Step 1 - Do

Step 2 - Un-do

Step 3 - Paws. Oops, pause.

That's it. This secret formula is how we take care of the pains, strains and struggles and relieve our muscles, refresh the movement system and return back to comfort.

Now let's dive a little deeper into the 3 steps and learn some of the keys to your success.

Step 1 - The Do

You can choose to either do the movement or imagine the movement taking place. Your brain will turn on the necessary and also unnecessary muscles which can initially substitute.

Our movement and programmed habits will turn up the volume so the muscles will go to work—and some of those that ideally could turn on, won't. This is partially why we're in the state we're in.

Your job, should you choose to accept the assignment, is to pay attention to whatever muscles or areas are turning on.

The feel and quality of a movement may seem vague when we haven't done a certain movement pattern in some time.

If things are initially unclear, this is OK. Thomas Hanna had a term called sensory-motor amnesia, wherein certain muscles have forgotten to do their job as others have taken over.

No worries, your brain will sort things out.

The Keys of the Do

1) Move slowly and with the least amount of effort.

This part is one of the hardest concepts to get since so many of us are used to turning things on with more effort than is necessary, otherwise our muscles would be more fluid, wouldn't you agree?

You'll be going through a phase of un-learning how to give so much effort and learning what the comfortable level of effort will be for you.

2) When necessary, do not move.

If you bump into pain, discomfort, or feel yourself straining too much, it's time to dial things down. Remember to move ever so gently, even to the point of imagining the movement if pain or discomfort emerges. Sometimes the hint of a movement can be enough to trigger a painful response. I know; I've tweaked myself enough times and have learned this lesson s-l-o-w-l-y over time.

3) Do what is necessary to be comfortable.

Find whatever props you need, such as a towel, pillow, cushion, roll of paper towels, etc. Place whatever materials you prefer underneath your body to make it as comfortable as possible. As your body returns to more comfort, then you can switch or change the props.

4) Modify to your heart's content.

Whatever the movement position is, say, for instance you're on your belly and, for whatever reason, on any particular day this is too painful, no worries. You can do the same movement in another plane or relationship with gravity. If the movement is to be done on your back, you can try it on your side. Do what you need to do to be comfortable. If that means you have to sit one out, just do or imagine the movement from the sitting position.

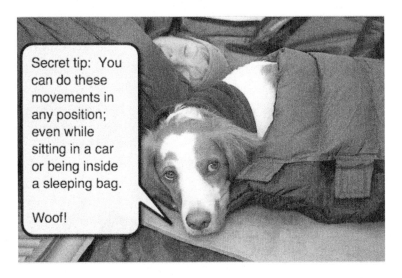

Secret tip: You can do these movements in any position; even while sitting in a car or being inside a sleeping bag.

Woof!

5) Go at your own pace.

There is no keeping up as this, in all likelihood, keeps things revved up. Even though in this "do" step you are revving up certain muscles; you are revving up them up to the degree in which you can be most comfortable doing or imagining so. You can rest as often as you need to.

6) Gaining length.

By keeping the movements smaller rather than larger, slower instead of faster, you'll regain muscular length more quickly. Go slow, get longer. Go fast, get tighter.

Step 2 The Un-Do

Wherever you end the movement, s-l-o-w-l-y back away and return to the place where you started from. As tension levels reset, this place may shift a little.

This step is the most important step to reset tension levels back to comfort.

Often times, this is the hardest one to perfect since we are so used to doing physical activity quickly which engages the brain's cerebellum. Normally, we'll want to undo a movement just as quickly since we got 'er done.

To get the motor cortex involved, we back away s-l-o-w-l-y.

In the un-doing of a movement you feel yourself as much as possible by noticing any changes in all or as many of the physical actions taking place.

When we do a movement, we may not necessarily feel all the actions and muscles that are involved. Things get clearer when we un-do a movement.

We'll begin to notice which muscles we are using, which ones are part of the entire movement, as well as feel certain actions and counterbalancing measures our brain's cerebellum will do for us.

How wide or narrow we want to focus our attention on the intention of the "do" part lets the un-do part serve notice as to what physical actions took place.

As certain tension levels decrease, we may notice other muscles or other parts of ourselves engaging or not engaging as much. We may wonder if certain actions are necessary to the "do" part in the first place.

The Keys of the Un-Do

1) Move s-l-o-w-l-y out of or away from the intended movement done in the "do" step.

As mentioned above, this is the part which has confounded many exercisers "going" for it and looking for the payoff of doing more.

By slowing the release of the area you contacted, this gives the brain the chance to do the necessary resetting actions. When we carefully feel our way through this step, we gain further and deeper insight as to how much of ourselves is involved in even the simplest of movements.

Even if you only do a micro-movement or imagine a movement, plenty of disengaging actions can take place.

2) Slowing down the s-l-o-w.

Instead of doing full range of movements, you might think of this as doing movement in half-ranges of motion from the view point of the targeted muscle or area which requires the participation of many muscles.

By paying very close attention, certain hiccups, misfires, hesitations or a jerky quality can normally result. When you see an animal pandiculate, you'll often see a limb returning in a similar manner as the duck in the video.

For the human animal, we can use this and profit by noticing whatever misfires happen. The next time we do the movement, we can slow the slow un-do even more and notice if there are more or less hesitations as a result.

3) Regaining control.

By going slow, the internal renegotiation of motor control reasserts itself. You may also notice other areas of involvement and can begin to detune or fine tune your use of your muscles and movement system.

Are certain muscles necessary when you are un-doing a particular movement?

The way to know is to feel your way through it. With practice, you'll begin to feel muscles which just jump on board and act as if they need to be involved. At this point, you may begin to consciously let an area or muscle relax more than it normally does.

This type of helper can now quiet itself down. You may begin to discover that it isn't as necessary to the movement you are intending to do.

You'll also discover in the un-do different ways of watching yourself feel your way out of the do.

4) Fine tuning.

As your brain creates more relaxation, the muscles become quieter in the sense that they are less reactive. They are more relaxed and will not necessarily jump on board.

Then, by your will or intention, you can turn more or less or different parts of yourself on to discover other muscular movement connections. This is why people will ask, "What is the right way?" The simple answer is, there is none.

There is a more optimal way for you to reorganize. This is accomplished by doing the un-do slowly. How slow you wanna go, that's up to you.

5) Uncovering tension and stress patterns.

Here is where you'll self-discover which muscles or areas from any number of layers are playing the perplexing part of your life. Since we have some 17 layers of muscles to organize, as you reorganize one layer, another may surface to uncover work needed to soothe things out.

6) Err into correction.

As the hesitations and misfires normally happen when you attempt to self-correct, know that the brain is on your side to reset things back to neutral. This has been called homeostasis. The nervous system shifts from being revved up to being and feeling calmer.

When we learned to walk, we weebled and wobbled our way to learn balance. This natural rebalancing act can also leave you feeling different when you're done.

As you stand up and walk around after being reset, the feel of your new and updated self may seem different from the old way you've been using your muscles.

Many people have experienced the feeling of being a drunken sailor or the sense of coming off of a ship at sea for an extended time, experiencing these natural self-corrections.

Your brain and body will get used to this as you will be using yourself differently, otherwise the old programming, which keeps you locked up, won't change much.

Erring into correction and moving back into your more youthful, more svelte self may be a long forgotten memory. When this happens, you'll notice how the shifting has moved you to a more comfortable place. When that happens ... welcome back to your former happy pandiculating self!

Step 3 - Paws the pause

This step is many people's favorite part. All you gotta do is rest. Stop. Turn everything off and feel whatever sensations or feelings arise from the do and undo steps.

This step can be tricky if you're used to being the doer, a go getter, the caregiver, the one responsible for the entire world—you know who you are. A moment's rest can seem like a luxury you no longer have or make the necessary time for.

How's that working out for you? A momentary pause, or longer, is what it takes for us to sense or perceive sensations or feelings which may come up.

The Keys of the Paws

1) Rest a little more than you think necessary.

Often times, we just wanna get through with it and move onto the next. This isn't that sort of activity or exercise. Remember, this is the un-exercise method so you can undo the tension and unlock any stress in the muscles or movement system.

Resting for a moment may seem like an eternity for some of you. As you become more relaxed, this phase will become more delicious for your body. It's just a matter of time, experiencing yourself in a conscious "off" mode.

2) The reset button.

This is where it is at. The brain will be releasing certain chemicals leading to relaxation. As you lie there, you'll notice whatever comes up.

3) Feelings or sensations.

We might judge or place words on the feelings or sense perceptions which arise. Often times, we may not have the words for the experience. This is normal and OK. You can allow any feeling or sensation that bubbles up.

You aren't trying to do anything about it; just feel or notice.

Sometimes there will be zip, nada, nothing. This is normal too. Other times, a whole variety of feelings can arise.

Naturally we may try to suppress the ones we don't like. That's cool. As the brain keeps the relaxation pump flowing on, we may not be used to the cocktail brewing.

This might even upset us as we look for a certain feeling or way of being since we're so used to who we are and how we feel or where the pain always seems to be.

All well and good. Getting back to comfort is a process and your body-mind needs the time to sort it out and get used to finding its way back to neutral.

If you've been living in 5th gear most of the time, that's what you'll look for or notice. Why am I not in 5th right now? How do I stay that way? No worries, it's much easier to get back to 5th if you're idling more easily. This will help you get to 5th with a lesser energy cost so can you ride 5th for longer.

Re-lubricating your joints and softening the muscles can be a scary or uncertain facet when you're used to doing things in a certain way. Regaining muscle function helps you keep what you got, while at the same time improve the overall use of yourself.

Once a program is in the brain, you got it. Now with a newer program, you return to a more comfortable way to move your entire being around.

Now you can truly rev up and rev down comfortably.

4) Breathing.

Noticing how you breathe as you rest is important. When the breathing pump does kick in, you'll remember what movements opened certain parts of yourself.

One woman gave up her neti pot of 30 years, which she had been using to improve her breathing. All she had to do was move easily, pay attention to letting go and wait to feel what arose.

5) When to begin again.

Whenever you want to; you go at your own pace. If you rush it, the muscles may not have reset. Next time, slow it down some more, rest for a certain conscious moment. Then you can move on.

Recap

The 3 steps are quite simple.

Step 1 - Do.

Step 2 - Un-do.

Step 3 - Paws. Wait or pause.

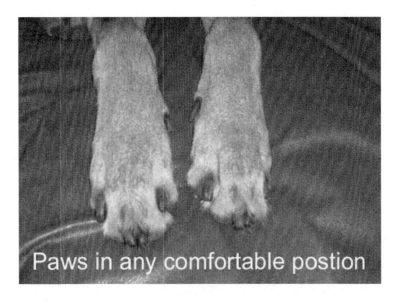

Paws in any comfortable postion

What is the 3 Step Method to Feel Comfortable,
be Flexible and Move Well for Life?

Remember, you don't have to do a movement, though you have to intend to do a movement. You either do it or imagine it. Then you slowly back off or imagine backing off while feeling what you can. Stop, rest and feel yourself.

In the following chapters, you're going to get to try the 3 step method for yourself with certain movement patterns. You'll get to understand how to unwind your own compensations and free up stiffness, high tension levels, stress or tightness, especially in the back or middle of yourself, namely the spine.

In the very next chapter, you'll get to do the key movement pattern which will serve as a bridge to all the rest of the system of pandiculations and somatics exercises. In no time, you'll move, reset and rest like a happy animal again.

Turn the page now to experience the key movement...

Chapter 5

What is the one Key Movement I can do to Feel Better Now?

In this chapter, you're going to get to do or imagine doing what I call the key movement pattern and bridge to the entire system of somatics exercises. You're going to understand the breakdown of the movement sequence and what to look for, feel and what you can possibly sense.

This movement pattern is vitally important to both wake-up the brain and body to set up comfortable movement for the entire day.

By using the 3 step method of a pandiculation, moving yourself in a certain direction, feeling the quality of the movement and its release, and allowing the brain to reset, you'll have completed one entire act of a pandiculation.

When you set your attention on the intention of a movement sequence or pandiculation from beginning to its return, your mindfulness and feelings of connection arise.

This promotes the feelings of well-being which allows us to move comfortably for life.

The Center of Gravity

In many movement traditions, the center of gravity is considered vital to being able to move with power, grace, ease and to be in control.

When we live with the ideal alignment, the center is often considered to be at the second sacral joint, S2 for short.

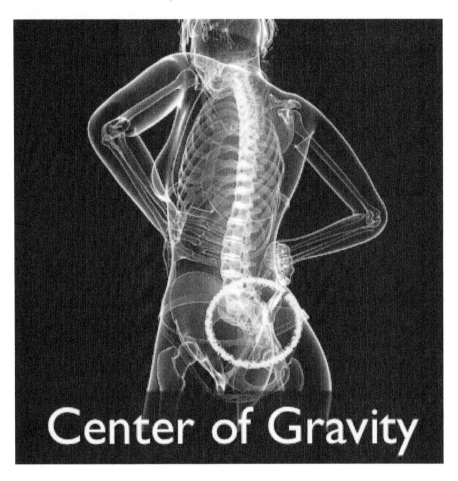

Since many of us hold any number of the compensations we talked about in chapters 2 and 3, our center can effectively be displaced either too low or too high and to the side as we trudge, teeter-totter, or heave ourselves about.

Even if we are an athlete with remarkable abilities, we can cheat in order to move as well as we can. We can still win medals with a few dysfunctions. The price we pay may end up as wearing out a joint, living with constant aches and having trouble recovering or lowering any tension and stress we accumulate from our activities.

For the brain and body to work cohesively and more easily, the flow of information from the brain out to the muscles and back can be improved with a spine that can move freely in a number of directions.

Core Mobility & Agility

Instead of the concept of core strength, you can consider core mobility and agility in order to regain control. The more the spine is able to be free in order to bend forwards, backwards, to the side and twist comfortably without being excessive, the more we can restore comfort and the sense of well-being from the middle outwards.

When the middle of our self is freer, then the more outward parts of our self, such as our legs, arms and head, can slide, glide, bend and turn in comfort.

This happens as the tension levels in the middle are less and are restored to neutral.

As tension levels diminish, we are also fine-tuning our senses and quality of movement itself. When we don't pay attention to this, we begin the slow ride to demise and that horrible sounding word, 'decrepitude', where the spring chickens won't ever return to the barn.

To refresh the nervous system, we wake-up our nervous system and body with a simple movement pattern. The brain's cerebrospinal fluid gets a chance to move and that noggin' of yours can ready itself for another day.

In the key movement pattern, the target will be the center of gravity. Once you re-establish the target and move with your intention, you'll be able to pick up more sensory information. Our proprioceptors come back online.

In the same way we've learned to update our computers, lest they get bogged down, we're simply updating our movement software to reboot, refresh and maintain itself.

As you focus on the middle, you'll be able to expand outwards, downwards and upwards and throughout your entire body. You shine your own flashlight of awareness on your movement system.

The flashlight will give you information on how things are moving or not moving, how stiff or easy, how comfortable or not ... and what may need a little more attention on any given day.

The key movement pattern is a different version often seen in many yoga classes called the cat-cow or cat-dog stretch. Instead of being on hands and knees, you'll begin on the floor or ground while lying on your back.

If that isn't comfortable, then you can adjust to lying on your side (knees atop one another) or using whatever pillows, towels or props are necessary to keep comfortable.

Why Range of Motion is Not the Deal?

Our emphasis will be different since you are tuning into the feelings, sense perceptions and quality of movement itself rather than how far or little you move. The range of motion isn't as important as the quality and your ability to move freely and comfortably in whichever range you have control.

Given your set of compensations or set of circumstances, one part of the following movement sequence may be easier or more of a struggle in terms of the 2nd part of the 3 step method.

When you let go of the intended direction, if there is a more hesitant or jerky quality, then this is the side of the equation or movement you'll need to spend a little more time with regaining control.

When this happens, remember the unconscious pre-programmed cerebellum is doing its job. Its set points are established. When you follow along, using your brain's cortex, you'll soon enough re-establish control and lower tension set points.

The Simple Key Movement Pattern

The spine will need to be reminded to extend itself by arching the back, following that with the slow release and the feel of how it lets go and what you can sense is involved. The other side of the coin is to flex the spine so it can round the back followed by paying attention to which muscles are releasing as a result of backing the back out slowly.

In the course of this simple exploration, you'll focus on your center of gravity and then you'll broaden the flashlight outwards, downwards and upwards.

Where to Start

Position: On your back with legs extended or knees bent. Lie in the most comfortable position for about a minute.

Feeling: Notice or feel whatever feelings or sense perceptions arise as you lie on your back.

Using whatever props you need, place a towel, blanket, or cushion underneath your neck, behind your head, under your hips, arms, etc. Whatever you need, make yourself as comfortable as possible.

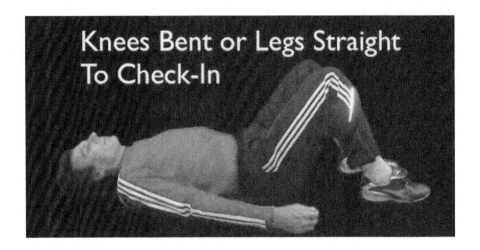

Simply lie on your back and, for a minute or so, feel what kind of contact you are making with the ground or surface. This is important to sense as a starting point of noticing and feeling whatever you can in this moment.

Once you've taken the vital time to sense how your body is presently making contact, now it is time to begin the actual movement series.

Recap the 3 Step Method & 1st Movement

Step 1 - Do.

Be as conscious as possible about your intention to move in the suggested direction as you move with the least effort. You can imagine this movement if it is too difficult to do.

Position: Bend your knees so your feet are flat.

Feeling: Zone into your center of gravity, near the S2 joint.

Do: You'll slowly extend the spine by arching your back slightly.

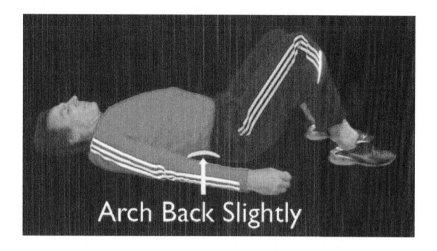

Arch Back Slightly

Feeling: What or where in your back are you contracting?

What other parts of yourself are involved as you arch the back a little?

Did you feel the sacral area of yourself moving? Could you sense how the tailbone moved in a downwards, or back- towards-the-ground, direction?

Do: On your next attempt, as you focus your attention on your sacrum, inhale and arch your back.

Feeling: Notice if the sacrum moves. Can you feel the area you are contracting or tensing in your lower back move forwards, relative to lying on the ground? Or did you brace with your belly and "try" to move the spine forwards?

This all depends upon your set of circumstances and habits of movement. If you're lying on your side, did you sense your spine in the lower back moving forwards? You can always try lying on your side and feel what happens.

The *key is the intention to move* in the suggested direction while attempting to arch the back.

49

When you zone in on the feelings of the contraction or tension, does it happen on both sides of your spine? Does one side tighten or contract more than the other? Or did you not notice the back contracting?

Step 2 - Undo.

Allow for the release to occur slowly, or imagine the releasing taking place if you imagined doing the movement.

After you've arched or contracted the lower back, you begin step 2 by s-l-o-w-l-y letting go.

Feeling: Feel if the action of letting go slowly is hesitant, jerky or smooth.

Step 3 - Paws or Stop.

Let the spine rest where it wants to.

Bring in Some Air

Do: As you begin to arch your back, inhale and let some air in.

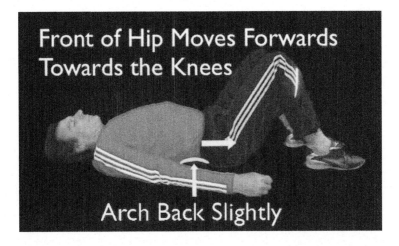

Feeling: As you begin to move and breathe in, notice if your pelvis or hip bones begin to move. Does the front top of your hips move forwards or downwards relative to your position?

Undo: Release the contraction or tension of your back.

Feeling: Do you get the sense your pelvis or hip bones roll back as you let the air out?

Paws. Then you wait as you rest for a moment.

For some of you, this may seem like a lot of information to keep up with, especially if you've been unconscious or proprioceptively illiterate. In other words, you may not have been paying attention to the position of your joints, the quality of movement itself and the associated feelings other than the discomforts you may be aware of.

No worries, your brain and conscious awareness can begin to check back in on the road to regaining control and self-adjusting for a comfortable life.

Next Repetition

Do: As you breathe in, move your sacrum to a comfortable point, and roll the pelvis as easily as you can.

Feeling: Feel if the back contracts or tenses.

Undo: Now you allow for the release of those efforts to occur.

Paws. Then you rest for a moment and lie there noticing any lingering sensations.

The Other Side of the Coin

Now that you've had the experience of extending the spine, you'll get to pay attention to the quality of flexing your spine. This is similar to curling into yourself, as if you're withdrawing to protect the front part of your body.

Position: Lying on your back, with your knees bent, feet flat (modify if lying on side).

Focus your attention on the middle of your body and the center of gravity.

Do: As you breathe out or exhale, pull your back into the surface or ground.

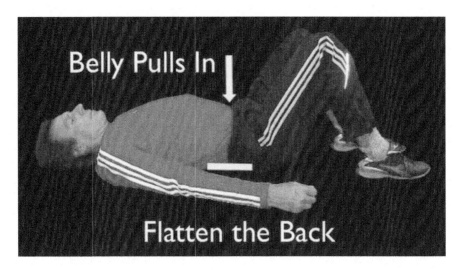

Feeling: Did your stomach muscles contract? Did you feel your belly move inwards?

Did your tailbone lift slightly? Were you able to keep your hips on the ground without lifting your buttocks up off of the ground?

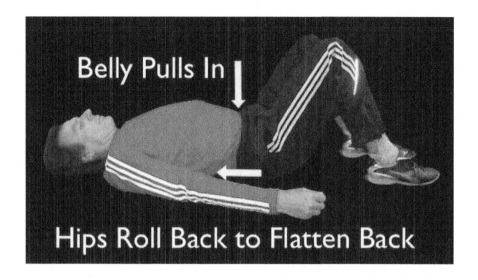

Belly Pulls In

Hips Roll Back to Flatten Back

You're merely rolling the pelvis or hip bones back or having the feeling of tucking them under so the spine may get the sense of flattening along the surface.

Your back is controlled from the front by those muscles in the belly. The abdominal muscles can contract to allow the back to flatten. Other muscles can participate as well, which you can discover as you practice.

The key is the letting go or step 2 un-do of the slow release.

Whatever contractions you used to pull yourself back, you can begin to pay attention to how you let them go. How smooth or jerky is the quality of the release?

Paws. Then, after you have released your back, you let the spine or back settle where it wants to. Rest for a moment.

Do: Take in a breath or two, begin again. Exhale and gently pull back the back.

Feeling: Focus on the contraction in your belly; it may or may not happen. Notice if the tailbone acts to lift slightly.

Undo: S-l-o-w-l-y release those actions.

Feeling: Notice what happens in the slow release.

As you release, you may notice the feeling of wanting to breathe in again. Go ahead and do so.

If your breath is too short, ideally begin breathing where you are at. Another key is to keep breathing as you are moving.

Do: On the next attempt, ideally as you exhale, you roll the pelvis or hip bones back, contract the stomach and flatten the back, feeling the tailbone or the bottom of the sacrum lifting slightly while keeping the back on the ground.

Undo: As you release, pay attention to how well you let go and the breath returning.

Paws. Then you rest. Take as long as you'd like.

More Optimal

Now that you've done the two parts of the coin, or movement sequence, you're going to combine and broaden your perspective.

It's one thing to be able to do or imagine the movement sequence.

Initially, you're interested in what the pattern is. You may be thinking, *Am I doing this right? I wish there was a video to see if I'm getting it.*

Since you're targeting a specific part of the brain, your brain's visual part is not involved.

The good news is there is no wrong way or right way to do these movements. There is, however, a more optimal and less optimal way to go about them.

The more optimal way will allow you to free up the nervous system so the lines of communication are clearer as you regain and improve the functions of your movement system.

The less optimal way brings up the discomforts we experience, creates greater pain and keep us stiff or more contracted rather than freeing up the restrictions which hamper our felt sense of freedom.

When we strain, force or push it too far, this goes against the notion of moving simply and easily. If you err, err on the side of moving or doing less and feeling as much as you can with as little movement as possible.

A micro-movement is better than a larger movement so you can remain well within your comfort zone.

As you regain control, then your range will naturally and comfortably increase.

To See or Not to See

While you may want to watch a video, this interferes with the part of the brain you are accessing. It's this part of the brain which can release the powerful chemicals of relaxation. So no worries, getting to know yourself all over again is both art and self-knowledge which will serve you for a comfortable lifetime.

As in all good learning, the process builds upon a foundation at first done s-l-o-w-l-y. The good news is that you're revisiting your ability to self-regulate your movement system. At some point in your life, the movement software was being updated. Now you're rebooting, refreshing and renewing the lines of information and communication along the feedback loop we talked about in chapter 2.

In time, you'll get better at resetting your own nervous system, just like all our fellow vertebrate animals who maintain their smooth moves simply through the act of pandiculation.

We're fortunate because we get to use our cortex systematically to unwind all the stresses and tensions we accumulate over a lifetime and on any given day. To age is to accumulate issues in the tissues. To age comfortably is set up by the natural act of pandiculation where we can figure out how to un-compensate and restore function simultaneously.

More Connections

Now that you have the idea of the movement pattern, you'll get to focus your attention more outwardly, relative to the middle of yourself.

Position: Begin again by lying on your back, knees bent, feet flat.

Do: As you breathe in, arch your back.

Feeling: Notice how your belly rises towards the ceiling. As you feel what is contracting and moving, what do you feel happening or taking place in your feet as a result of extending your spine or arching your lower back?

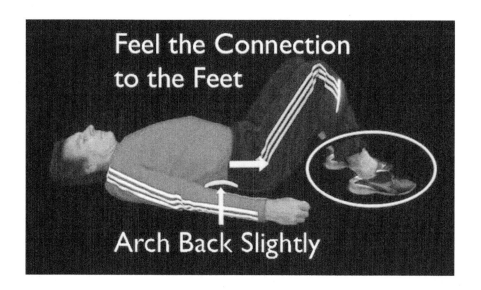

Undo: Exhale and release yourself. Give yourself the necessary slow time.

Feeling: Notice what is letting go once the spine or back has settled and you've taken the time to breathe in.

Do: You can begin to exhale and roll back the back.

Feeling: Notice the sensations underneath your feet.

Does it feel the same as when you arched your back or is there a slightly different feeling in your feet as you move the back back?

Undo: Notice how well you release.

Feeling: What releases as you pay attention to the quality of coming back to where you started?

Paws. Come to a complete rest.

Repeat the entire 2 part pattern, in this 3 step graduated manner.

Do: Breathe in and arch your back.

Feeling: Feel your feet.

Undo: As you slowly release, allow the air to let go too.

Paws. Then a brief rest.

Do: Actively breathe out, roll the pelvis back.

Feeling: Notice how your feet respond to the movement in the middle of yourself.

Undo: Once again, slowly release and come to a rest.

Now go ahead on your own and redo the entire sequence and pay attention to how your feet respond as you focus your attention on the middle of yourself.

After you've completed the movement, rest. Tune into any lingering feelings or sensations as they arise or come up.

By tuning in, you may be getting a sense of the chemicals of relaxation you've created. By shifting the nervous system to a more relaxed state, your sense of it may cause a yawn to occur. Other pleasant sensations may arise.

You may feel that your position on the floor has changed or the ground has become more comfortable. You may feel heavier or lighter. You may feel the blood flowing or energy or words that cannot describe or pinpoint the feelings you are sensing.

Any number of sense perceptions or feelings can occur.

If you pushed yourself, the other side of the nervous system may have been turned on and you can feel the reverse of the more pleasurable feelings.

Shifting Gears

Now you'll shift your attention to the other side of yourself, namely the head end or top of yourself.

Do: Inhale and arch your back.

Feeling: Notice what you do about your head.

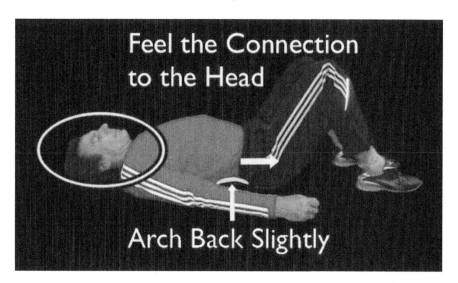

Does your head lie still or does it move with you as you move your spine?

Undo: Release and let go of the contraction in your spine.

Feeling: Does the head slightly move or remain still?

Paws.

Do: Consciously exhale and gently round your lower back.

Feeling: Does your head move? Does it move similarly to the previous movement or does it feel as though it is moving forward? Does it roll off to one side? Is it rigidly adhering to the ground?

Undo: As you release your stomach muscles, your spine releases and your head releases. Allow all the parts of yourself to settle where they want to.

Paws. As you rest, notice again any lingering sensations.

Now go through the entire sequence.

Do: Inhale and arch your back.

Feeling: Notice what the arching of your back does to your head.

Undo: Slowly release.

Feeling: Notice if there is a slight movement in your head.

Paws.

Do: Actively exhale and move in the opposite direction.

Feeling: How does the head play along with the movement?

Undo: Slowly release.

Feeling: How does the head move?

Repeat the cycle.

Do: Inhale and arch your back and allow your head to freely move.

Feeling: Notice what happens to your chest and shoulders.

Do you get the sense your shoulders are falling back or moving forwards?

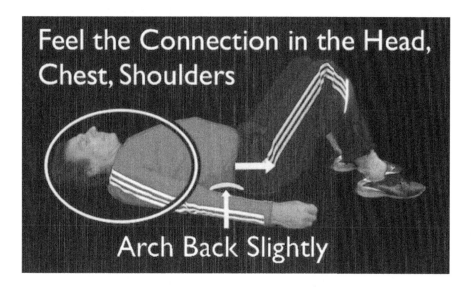

Undo: Allow for the release.

Paws for a brief momentary pause.

Do: Consciously begin the exhalation and contraction of the belly and lifting of the tailbone.

Feeling: Does your head move or not? What is happening in your shoulders or chest? Do your shoulders feel as if they're moving forwards or are they not moving in conjunction with the movement of the middle of yourself?

Undo: Then pleasantly allow for the release of all of the actions.

Paws.

Repeat the entire sequence and notice the movement of your head, the feelings in your chest, in your shoulders... Then, as you release, reverse course until you release and rest once again.

Paws for as long as you'd like.

Do and Undo: Now you're going to repeat the same pattern of inhaling and arching your back by zoning into the center of gravity and allowing that to release. Then you'll actively exhale and flatten the back and release.

Feeling: As you repeat, pay attention not only to your head; feel what is happening with your feet. Notice the feelings or movement in your arms or legs.

Now you're broadening out your perspective as you notice the other parts of yourself.

Repeat the entire do and undo.

What is happening with your feet?
What is happening with your head?
What is happening with your arms?
What is happening with your legs?

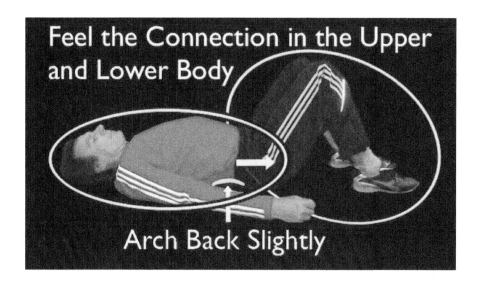

Are things feeling tight or rigid, or is your intention to move your middle, the center of gravity, affecting the rest of you?

Notice how your body naturally responds without imposing any response to it.

Repeat the do and undo.

As you reverse your course, do things move opposite, or in the reverse, direction?

As you release, what is it that is releasing, what gives, how well does it let go; can you release it more smoothly each time?

Big paws. Then turn off and rest all of your efforts.

As you lie there, tune into any feelings or sense perceptions that you are aware of in this moment.

Give yourself all the time you need to linger ...in whatever it is you are aware of.

Did your relationship with the floor change?

What do you notice about your breathing?

Do you feel more relaxed?

Did you yawn at some point?

Do you feel lighter, heavier, grounded, more solid, more connected, springier?

Is there no feeling at all?

Sensory Motor Connections

All of this is sensory information. As you begin to practice and reacquaint yourself with the mindful act of pandiculation, then you become aware of motorizing a movement—initiating from the brain's cortex with your intention to move in a certain direction.

You are reminding the muscles of their function and the connections they make; corresponding to the feelings associated with a certain movement pattern or place in space.

This is what we can redevelop, re-establish and re-coordinate along the entire chain of the movement sequence.

By focusing on the center of gravity, you notice what you can, even if you stay in the small window at the center of gravity. You can scale things up and down, as you got to experience here, or you can refocus on certain parts of yourself as to how they relate to the intention to move a certain part.

Now go ahead and do the movement sequence again a few times and compare this to when you first did the movement, when you zoned in on the center of gravity.

How does the quality of your movement feel now?

Remember this is not about the range of motion, it's about how and what you feel in the simple journey of extending and flexing your spine. To regain control is to know certain aspects along this movement continuum.

Now you've experienced the key somatics movement. This movement serves as the bridge to the entire system of somatics exercises.

You're going to revisit this pattern as we add in the game changer of differentiation in the next few chapters.

This will begin the process of de-compensating held postures, misalignments and dysfunction, relieve stress and high tension patterns on your way to feeling freer and less stiff, simply by freeing up the middle and working outwards to our periphery.

Recap

You got to do the 3 step method of pandiculation using the key somatics exercise pattern which is a bridge to the system of movements to help keep us free so we can move like an animal again and again.

In the next chapter, we're going to cover what is happening more commonly these days, the kinds of postures we're seeing in terms of the signs of our times. If you find yourself too stiff from sitting, the next chapter will help. If you want to skip ahead to our Wanna Move

Faster—Go Getter chapter 7, by all means, the moves are in there to help you get all you want. The following chapter 8 has a wonderful sequence to deal with the blows, traumas and falls we've racked up in our lifetime.

OK, to find out what those handheld devices, sitting too much and other scary, frightening events do to our bodies so that we lose our animal sense of moving well, turn the page.

Chapter 6

Stiff from Sitting?

In this chapter we're going to take the 2nd part of the key movement pattern a little further with a different, broader and deeper way to experience it so we can sit more comfortably.

Do you feel stiff when you've been sitting for some time? Do you dread a long car ride? Do you have to groan to get up? Are you using your hands to push down to get up from sitting?

Sitting for too long has proven to be not in our best interests. We'll tend to stiffen. Even regular exercise cannot counteract the number of hours many of us sit.

Certain circumstances in life cause us to withdraw, fold inwards, or sink into ourself. Ever had a bad day and feel the need to curl into yourself? This normal act or movement happens in times of trauma as if someone punched us in the gut.

How We Adapt

You may be in an occupation or activity sitting for a length of time. Gravity begins to bear down upon us causing us to sink further.

Today's toys of checking the email or the more urgent text message, and playing video games while hunching over where we bend our arms and crane our head to see the "important" information in our lives forms a repeated posture.

When we think of our arms being bent while driving a car, sitting at a computer, emailing, the act of eating. Any number of things we do, we can see how our shoulders have adapted.

Take a look in any grocery store and watch people walk and see how many palms are facing backwards on account of shoulders rolling forwards.

When arms are in neutral, they tend to face each other. When shoulders are rounding on account of the hours we spend doing certain activities like typing on a keyboard which puts our hands (palms) facing backwards.

If only we had keyboards where we'd type upside down, then our shoulders would normally fall back rather than being pulled forwards.

Feelings

When we experience feelings of worry or anxiety, we can begin to see how our body adapts and molds itself around these experiences too. Certain patterns begin to manifest over time.

When we're apprehensive, we may have the tendency to withdraw into ourself. Much in the same way a scared animal withdraws to protect itself. Our spines respond in a similar protective manner.

We round or flex the spine causing the chest to sink down. Our shoulders may move forward in response.

Gravity Wins

A typical posture of seeing someone with a stomach sinking in, a chest depressing and a head lurching forwards. This kind of posture when we're engaged while sinking in resembles the pattern when we get startled.

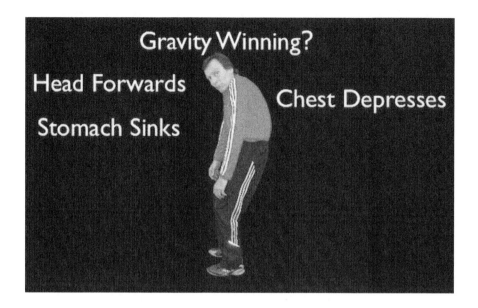

As we age, the common thought is well, this is what happens. Gravity gets the best of us. All the build up of the pressures, demands, anxieties and the fears we feel accumulate.

When we have the feeling of losing, we normally sink. The opposite is winning where we tend to rise up with our chest. When we sink, the chest moves downwards.

Even the people who read with their knees-knocked and obviously arms bent are unconsciously bringing the chest wall downwards. This default posture may result from any number of circumstances and can feel normal over time.

If someone is saying things we don't like, we might bring our legs in and cross them or hold them tighter together without consciously knowing it. And we can even adapt to keeping our arms crossed as a go to.

Our everyday experiences and the ways we hold ourself together accumulate in our tissues. When certain patterns keep playing themselves over and over, our tissues begin to protest.

How Do We Take Care Of Sinking In?

Our muscle viewpoint is to strengthen that which is pulling us downwards. We attempt to do the opposite. How many times did we hear or have to say, sit up straight.

By attempting to strengthen a so called slack back this should offset the pull from the muscles of the front which are usually plenty strong from repeatedly being used.

The repeated habit of being pulled in or downwards, keeps the message repeating to keep things taught, tight and tensed. The muscles respond to the position and we lose another battle to the proprioceptive police. The arrests continue in our self-imposed prison of immobility and lack of freedom in movement though it can feel normal once we've adapted long enough in it.

When we understand the signal from the brain is held "on" to pull us inwards, downwards or sinking in, we can use that to set ourselves free rather than strengthen ourself to brace against the signal which would still be kept on.

By pandiculating, we can turn off or tune down that "on" signal, so our spine can freely move upwards and not be held sinking down.

Keeping the Spine Flexed

Some people like to sleep with 2 or 3 pillows propped up underneath them. If you remove the pillows, then things could be uncomfortable. This is usually a sign of someone who would rather sleep or be positioned in the more curled in manner.

This keeps the spine in a more flexed position as we can adapt ourself to positions where the muscles shorten and in time this feels normal to us.

The only problem with this kind of normal, no matter if you still possess a wonderful spirit, is the limitation of movement and inability to move as freely as you once did.

Lying in a variety of positions is more beneficial for the long run rather than lying in the same position when you go to sleep.

Moving in Your Comfort Zone

When doing any of the self-corrective movement patterns initially, it is far wiser to work within your comfort zone so having the prop of pillows as you need them is OK for starters.

In time as your spine loses the held tension, then you may lose one level of a prop and eventually return the spine to a more neutral and normal lengthened position.

In the same manner you've seen a cat luxuriously lengthen itself, we too can get back those cat like feelings of lying long.

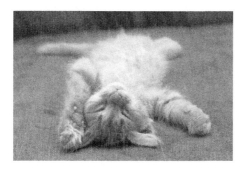

Back to the Key Movement

In the second part of the key movement, where you flexed your spine so your back went back, you got a glimpse of what you're about to experience.

Even while you're seated, you can focus on the center at gravity at S2, the second sacral joint. Move the sacrum back, this will cause the spine to flex back and the chest to move in a downwards direction.

Use What is On Instead

If you find yourself sitting or feeling slumped, instead of trying to straighten yourself up, you'd begin by slumping yourself more. This turns on more of what your body is currently doing.

Then you can allow yourself to release out of the slump so you can more easily sit upright without trying to hold yourself upright.

Once again, this is reverse to many approaches since you are releasing a held tension pattern. Go with the on signal, in order to turn it off. Then "on" will turn "off" more easily.

The Best Chair

When the spine is more functional, the tension on all sides is more equal so sitting without a back support or back of a chair is easy. This is the more normal healthy state of things since the best chair we have is our own two legs and a healthy spine.

Yet how many of us have lost the ability to comfortably squat, sit crossed legged or sit on our heels as we age.

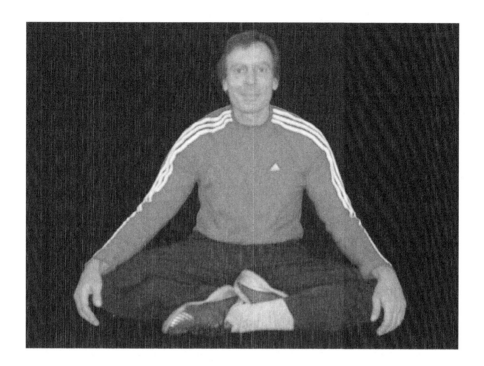

Personally I've had to keep playing movement games to maintain these abilities since I get wrecked in the games I play and I have to put humpty-dumpty back together again.

Having the knowledge of the tools is half the fun. Getting to experience this over and over as I age, I marvel and revel in the extraordinary exquisiteness of renewal. I ask myself if there is anything else I'd rather be doing than recreating the amazing feelings coursing through my body. As a child we didn't want to miss our chance to play. As an adult, we can keep on renewing and enjoying our physical pursuits.

Today, when people are sore, tired, stiff and more immobile than they care for, the better option seems to be to miss an event or activity. Hopefully, we're taking the time to get back on track with a useful set of tools we can rely on to improve.

The Next Movement Pattern

This new movement pattern will be broken down into manageable parts so at the end you put the entire movement together.

Just like the initial key movement pattern, you'll first learn to get the hang of the movement, then we'll broaden the perspective so you sense and feel the connections.

Remember if you don't feel or sense the connections, it just means the lines of communication aren't clear. With your *intention* to move, eventually the weeds clear out and the lines of information become clearer.

You'll sharpen your focus as initially things may fire all over the place.

When we get startled, typically our chest depresses, shoulders round up, the stomach sinks and our head lurches forwards, and we withdraw our legs and arms to protect ourself in the moment.

We can use this experience of withdrawing into ourself. We can feel what is taking place so when or if it happens for too long or to our detriment, we can use this knowledge to comfortably move out of this "on" or holding pattern.

The Moves to Set Us Free to Begin to Sit More Easily

Position: Begin by lying on your back, knees bent, feet flat, arms along or near your sides.

If you need pillows to prop your back, legs, feet... whatever the case, make yourself comfortable. In time as you regain mobility and get more comfortable, the props can go away.

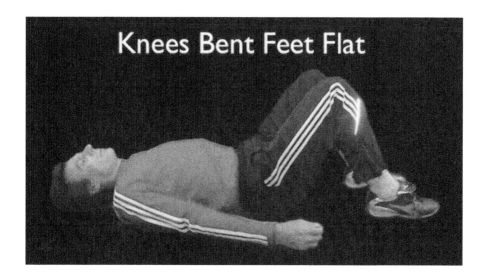

You'll begin first with a warm-up of doing the 2nd part of the key movement pattern.

Remember the 3 step method. Do, Undo, Paws - stop or rest.

Do: Focus your attention on the center of gravity, around the sacrum. Exhale as you roll the pelvis or hips back causing the muscles of the belly to contract so the back flexes or moves into the surface as the tailbone slightly lifts or tucks under.

Feeling: Feel how this begins to pull the chest downwards.

Undo: Allow for the slow release.

Paws.

Do: Repeat the movement again.

Feeling: Notice if it feels as if your shoulders want to move forwards. In some cases, there may be no movement at all in the shoulder.

This happens when things are frozen or we tend to move like a block. Remember this is a normal adaptation even though it may not serve us for the long run.

The practice of mindful movement will eventually free the areas up when we differentiate micro-movements such as this one.

Do: Roll your pelvis back as you exhale and contract the belly.

Feeling: Notice if the shoulders move forward or the chest is moving downwards.

Undo: Allow for the slow release.

Paws.

A Step Further

Now you'll shift your focus to the head end of yourself.

When we almost shut our eyes, we can make those crows eyes.

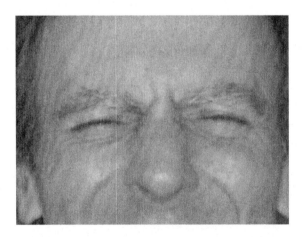

Do: Squinch your eyes so you can create those crows eyes while at the same time tightening your jaw by opening your mouth comfortably wide.

Feeling: Notice if your shoulders feel as if they rise up ever so slightly.

Undo: Slowly release.

Sensing: Did you sense any movement in the shoulders? If you did, good, if you didn't...

Do: Repeat by squinching the eyes, tightening the jaw and micro-move, i.e. barely lift the shoulder or allows the shoulders to lift in response.

Feeling: Did you get a sense your chin acted to lift up or move forward slightly?

Undo: Slowly release.

Paws.

Do: Squinch your eyes, tighten the jaw, allow the shoulders to rise up (towards the ceiling) and let the chin tilt up slightly.

Undo: Slowly release.

Repeat the movement.

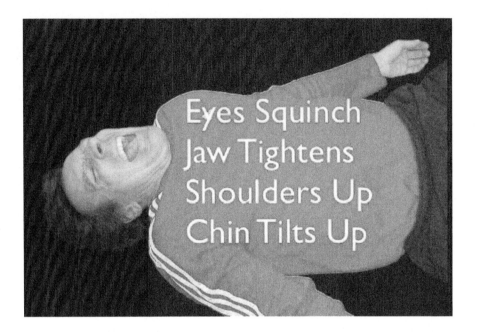

Feeling: Did you notice how your chest is beginning to sink?

Do: Repeat and exhale or breathe out easily.

Undo: As you release, allow your breath to come back in.

Paws again.

Do: With your next exhalation. Squinch the eyes, tighten the jaw, allow the shoulders to rise, let the chin lift up slightly, let the chest sink down and now bring in the 2nd part of the key movement by rolling the pelvis back and contracting the belly.

Feeling: Did you curl further into yourself? Did your chest sink a little lower?

Undo: Release slowly.

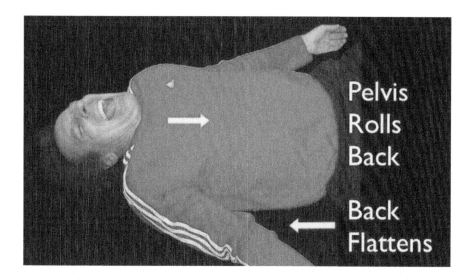

Feeling: Notice how artfully you can slowly let go.

If you had to protect yourself or your upper body say from a ball flying at you at high speed, you might choose to bring in the arms as a shield.

Do: Repeat as above, squinch the eyes, tighten the jaw, allow the shoulders to rise, let the chin lift, chest sinks down, contract the belly, roll the pelvis and now bend the arms and move them to your chest as you make a light fist while bending the wrists.

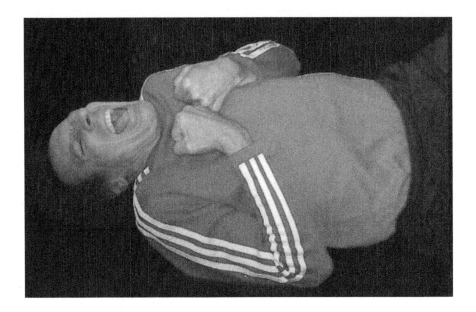

Feeling: Do you feel your shoulders wanting to move forwards or up towards the ceiling?

Undo: Slowly release the contractions and tension in your hands, arms, chest, belly, shoulders, neck and head.

Paws and then...

Do: Curl into yourself, squinting the eyes, tightening the jaw, raising the shoulders, arms bending in, wrists flexing, hands curling in, belly tightening, pelvis rolling back as the chest wall sinks downwards.

Undo: Release the feelings and tension pattern you created.

Feeling: How smooth can you release all the conscious tension patterns you created? Were any parts more sticky or stuck or hesitant to let go?

Paws once again.

Remember how I mentioned our idea of a bookworm, someone who reads with knocked-knees. Let's add this piece to the pattern.

Do: As you begin to exhale and contract all the parts of yourself in your upper and middle part of your body, bring the bent knees in towards each other.

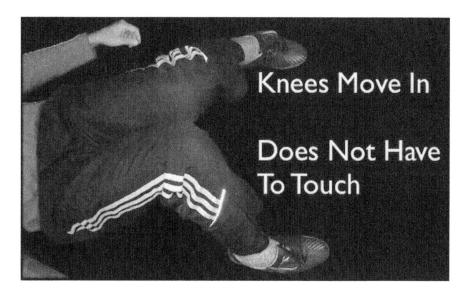

Feeling: Did this cause you to feel the chest sinking lower or curling further inwards?

Undo: Slowly release.

Paws. Take a few breaths and feel whatever sensations may arise at this moment.

Then, when you're ready:

Do: Repeat the entire sequence and as the legs move inwards, lift the toes by keeping the balls of the feet more on the surface.

Feeling: You may feel the front of the lower legs, the shin area begin to contract, tense or tighten along with all the other parts of yourself you are actively and mindfully engaging.

Now you have the fuller, broader and deeper effect and sense from toes to the head of what you can sense, feel or tense as we withdraw in one of the many ways we can.

Undo: And as always, release yourself slowly.

Feeling: What it is you are letting go of while coordinating the timing of letting go.

Paws. As you rest, allow the air to move in and out of you a few times.

Do: Repeat the entire pattern.

Feeling: As you protect your body and withdraw into yourself, moving gently, what is it that you move and sense with your conscious awareness? Where do you pull more? Where do you pull less?

Undo: As you release, you'll end up where you started in the neutral position.

Now that you've experienced yourself closing in. It's time to allow for an opening.

Do: As if you're doing a jumping jack, allow your arms to slowly slide away from your side as you allow the knees to drift apart (well within your comfort zone) as if you resemble a frog.

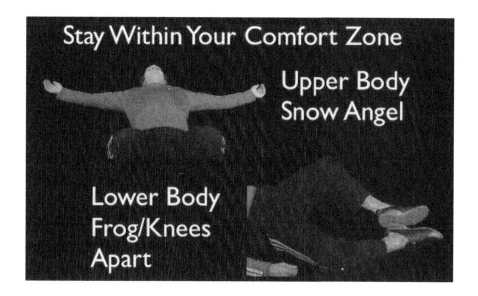

Feeling: Lie there for a moment and feel the open-ness and the exact opposite of being held or closed in. You can hang out there for as long as you'd like.

Undo: Slowly move yourself back into the neutral or starting position.

Big Paws.

Turn everything off and rest in place with either your knees bent or legs extended.

Feeling: As you lie there, notice and feel whatever sense perceptions or feelings arise as result from mindfully being aware of the movement you experienced.

Withdrawal Reflex

The withdrawal reflex is a normal set of physical actions where our body moves itself in response to being startled. As the danger is over, we normally begin to release this set of actions.

If the danger, fear, or difficult situations persists, our tissues soaks this information in. Now you have some moves to release this type of held reflex pattern which can creep in while we sit.

Ways to Counteract Too Much Sitting

The number of hours we sit for instance, where gravity exerts its toll, may not be countered by exercise. A simple key is to either get up as often as possible or become more present and mindful of sitting and how we can mindfully self-adjust even while sitting.

It is possible to sit and work comfortably for hours given enough mindful attention on the inner game of being proprioceptively aware. This can simply begin by doing what all healthy vertebrate animals do in the morning. Prepare the physical body by taking out the accrued muscle shortening which naturally happens overnight.

Then throughout the course of your day, self-correct as necessary.

Once you learn this particular pattern, you can re-create this while seated. You can always imagine yourself doing it too, lest your co-workers or fellow commuters are wondering what all the writhing is about. Naturally, you may be the one who offers to help them when their stiffness and tension patterns no longer abate.

You have the power and the ability to create chemicals of relaxation which provide the necessary reminder of certain muscular functions which will go away if not tended.

You either lose it or use it. The choice is clearly yours. This can be done following our intention of simple conscious movement. Whether we take the time to imagine the movements and releases taking place or we do a micro-movement which is barely perceptible, the update to our movement system occurs.

Recap

This particular pattern is helpful for those of us who live with rounded shoulders, a stooped posture, a sinking chest, an overly hardened belly, knocked knees, video gamers, being in a vehicle for a length of time or you happen to sit a lot.

This movement can serve as a beginning to free yourself up in the morning, during the day, and at night to free yourself from the accumulated tension or stress you took on.

For you wanna go faster—go getter types, the next chapter will serve you as the the next movement pattern will de-tune the holding or high tension levels and reinvigorate the body to help you keeping moving as fast as a cheetah.

Chapter 7

Wanna Move Faster?

A re you a go getter? Is your life on the go-go-go? You may not want to spend a lot of time taking care of yourself since there is so much to do. Do I got your number?

You're going to be able to change things fairly quickly. It is going to take a little bit of time to integrate the work your brain and body will do for you. Your brain will work immediately to reset the muscles and movement system to lower stress and tension levels when you follow the 3 step method you learned in chapter 4.

Quick as a Cheetah

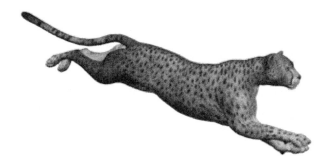

Have all the stress you want or that you can take on. Get all amped up, go with your gusto, rev things up. Be as quick as a cheetah. Then with a simple set of tools you can de-amp, re-tune and go back out there and "do" it again.

We know cheetahs aren't pulling their hamstrings running 60 mph on account of setting themselves up with their series of pandiculations. A reset here or there and you can go-go-go comfortably too.

A typical posture we tend to see with people who are on the go, ready to go, go, go.

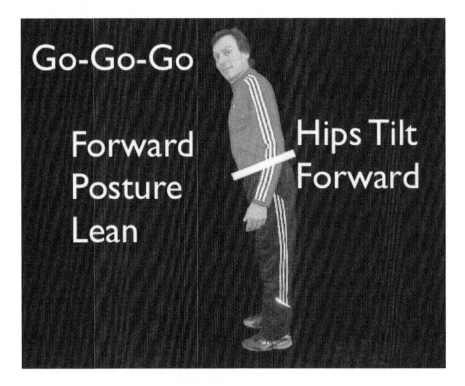

The pelvis or hips are tilted or rotated more forwards. The stereotypical beer gut kind of guy with a belly hanging forwards or a girl whose buttocks juts out and perhaps her legs are overextending or forwards of a standing plumb line. She is ready to go as is our beer drinker ready for the next watering hole with his pelvis rotated forwards.

The World of Exercise

In the exercise world, what we normally think to do is, «Well you gotta do more sit ups, ab crunches», so this can counteract and reshape the belly. You gotta do more core work so the pelvis or hips can move back in the more neutral position.

You gotta strengthen a weak front to offset the strong pull in the back since it takes some muscles being pulled forward by either the weight it has to counteract or the tension of the pattern being ready to go-go-go a majority of the time.

When we go to move forwards, the back contracts to ready us for action. Even our thoughts of our to-do list turns on certain readying muscles. If I'm thinking I gotta do this, there isn't enough time so I'll hurry things. Go-go-go and the back and readying muscles keep getting turned on.

The Animal World

With our animal approach to resetting all the go-go stuff we do, we can look at what the signals are programming us to do. Which is to hold the pelvis or hips tilted in a forwards or ready position so our back muscles are "on".

The message to keep contracting remains on. Instead of taking the muscular approach to reset or resolve matters, we're going to do the opposite by "working with" the signal and flow of information which is turned "on".

This seemingly counterintuitive approach is what all the healthy animals are doing.

We'll move ourself back into comfort by moving into the direction of the "on" signal rather than trying to create equal tension on the opposite side of the muscles.

Through your level of sensitivity coupled with your sense and quality of movement, you're going to be able to turn things "off" so the muscles come back to rest.

Your back will fall back and lose the gut or allow for the buttocks to drop down so the spine is no longer being tensionally held in the forwards or "on" position. Now it can truly let go and be able to turn on more easily and comfortably.

Regaining Control

When you begin to feel yourself getting overly amped or too tensed or tight, you merely lie down and do a few simple movements to take the tension and stress back out in order to regain control.

What do you need to know in order to regain control?

Just as we did in the previous 2 chapters, the movement patterns will be broken down into parts so you'll learn what to do and what to look for to sense or feel your way through the entire part of a particular pattern.

At the end, there will be a more global movement pattern you can do when you run out of time and need a quick fix. The parts of the pattern will serve you to facilitate different aspects of yourself. You'll be able to tune into similarities and notice differences as they arise.

Remember your comfort is your priority. Prop yourself as necessary with blankets, towels or cushions.

Go-Getter Movement

Position: You'll begin by lying down on your back with either your legs straight or knees bent with your arms comfortably lying down near or at your sides.

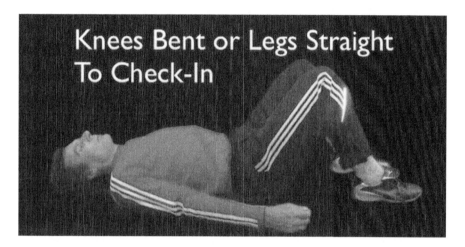

Feel how your body makes contact with the surface. Then after a minute, bend the knees so the feet are flat. This will be your starting position.

In the key movement pattern from chapter 5, where you learned about arching your back. This is where you'll begin as a go-getter.

Do: You'll begin with that simple part of breathing in. As you inhale, arch your lower back, so that your pelvis can roll forwards and your tailbone can tip slightly back.

Feeling: Tune into where you sense a contraction or tightening or tensing taking place in your back.

Undo: Allow for a s-l-o-w and controlled release.

Feeling: If you're a super go-getter, when you release, things will ratchet back, be hesitant, or have a jerky quality, or won't be as smooth as it could possibly be.

This is normal if you're feeling overly amped or a wee bit tight or the pelvis is rotated more forwards.

When you actively engage your movement system with your conscious awareness, by slowing things down, you dis-engage the tension pattern so the brain can do the reset.

Less Effort

Do: When you're ready, you'll move once again easily and gently using less effort. Move well within your comfort zone.

Feeling: Tune into what is contracting or tensing while you are moving.

This information may or may not be clear. That's OK. By doing the movement, you are contracting certain muscles and muscle groups.

Undo: Allow for the slow release.

Feeling: Notice if things begin to feel a little softer or more in your control with each release.

Paws.

A Key in the 3 Step Method

Remember you're a go-getter. You may feel like you just want to do the movement and get it over with. Remember the 3 step method of doing. Undoing is key. Giving yourself sufficient rest or a paws which lets the brain make the necessary changes.

The paws or rest may seem like an eternity to a go-getter because you want to get on with it. Well, you are getting on with it by resting. This allows the spine to fall back into a more neutral position. The momentary rest can be crucial since it will allow you to do your life at a faster pace. Now that you know how to reset tension levels back to neutral.

Do: Repeat the movement one more time easily, lightly, gently as you inhale and arch your back.

Feeling: What or where are you contracting? Is your pelvis rolling?

Remember in the first key movement how you paid attention to your feet and your shoulders.

Enlarge your picture of awareness or feel more broadly throughout your body.

Undo: Slowly release all of your efforts.

Feeling: Feel what is letting go. Allow your spine to settle into the surface.

Paws. Then take a moment to feel whatever lingering sensations or feelings you are aware of.

This is how you can start things to begin to de-amp and de-tune tension levels in the lower back.

Now you're going to do the next movement.

Position: On back, one knee bent, one leg straight.

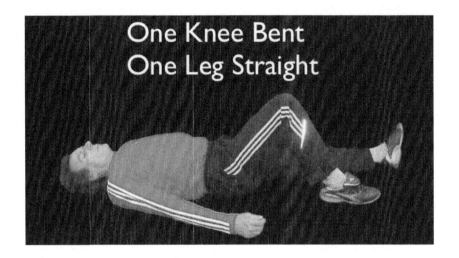

Do: On the bent leg side, allow the knee to drift out to the side as if it could move out towards the floor. Remain in your comfortable range.

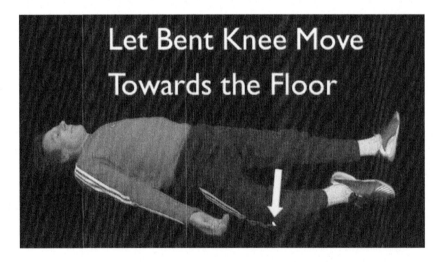

Undo: Slowly and easily bring the knee back up to where it started.

This movement is called external rotation. It's as if you are standing up, bending the knee and turning the knee outwards. Certain muscles will begin to engage when you actively do this movement.

94

Do: Turn the knee out to the side.

Undo: Slowly allow for the knee to travel back.

Feeling: If the undo is ratchety or hesitant This is information you can use the next time.

Paws.

Your job is to find a way to do it more smoothly. If you move out half as far, that's OK. Make sure you move in your comfort range as you attempt to regain control. This will come back with practice.

Do: Let the knee go out to the side.

If you're comfortable at this point, then you can be a little more active. Actively push the knee towards the floor or ground.

Feeling: You may feel other muscles turning on as you do this part a little more actively.

If this is well within your control and it feels comfortable, then by all means, you can do so.

Undo: Now the key is to s-l-o-w-l-y come back to the place where you started.

Paws and turn off all of your efforts. Slide the bent leg long.

Feeling: How does this side of yourself feels compared to the other side. How does your back feel? How do the feelings in the legs compare?

As you lie there, tune into whatever feelings or sense perceptions arise.

By lying there, you are still doing the work by not doing anything. Paying attention to what is going on whether you sense any information or not is part of the doing nothing or paws step. This fosters a different type of awareness.

Reposition: Bend the other leg.

Do: Allow the knee to drift out to the side.

Undo: Allow the knee to come back up.

Paws.

Then repeat the movement.

Feeling: Notice the quality of the movement. Does this side feel the same or a little different than the other side. Does the undo feel similar or different?

On the third and final attempt, if comfortable and you're capable, you can attempt to press the knee out closer towards the floor.

Undo: Slowly return. Bring the knee up towards neutral or where you started.

Paws. Turn everything off and come to a rest. Allow the bent leg to straighten.

Feeling: Notice qualitatively what this leg feels like.

If at any point straightening the legs is dis-comforting, then keep the knees bent and compare the legs in the knee bent position.

Position: Have both knees bent.

Do: Allow both knees to drift out away from each other.

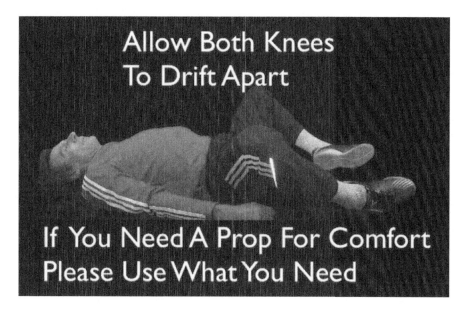

Undo: Bring the knees back in to where you started.

Paws.

This of course is opposite to what you learned in the previous chapter for the folks who are held more in or withdrawn. People that tend to be on the go are showing postures of more open-ness at the hips or feet splayed out like a duck.

Repeat the movement sequence.

When I see someone walking down the street with feet splayed wide, and the hips are swinging, this clues us into what could be happening with their pelvis and spine.

Do: Simultaneously, take both knees out to the side. Then gently press the knees out for a moment to feel or sense the contraction or tension in doing this part of the movement.

Feeling: Do you feel the outside of the buttocks contract? Do you feel the outside of your legs contracting? Does your back arch up more?

Undo: Slowly back away from that contraction or comfortable position you went towards. Slowly bring the knees back up to where you started.

Paws completely.

Feeling: Notice how you are breathing.

Let's add an inhalation to your next movement.

Do: As you inhale, lower both of your legs outwards.

If you need to take another breath by all means do so.

Then gently press the knees out (inhale again if you need to) towards the surface.

Undo: Slowly release the outward pressure as you exhale and begin to bring the knees back in.

If you need to take another breath, please do so.

Paws.

On the third and final attempt do the entire movement using the least amount of effort.

Feeling: Paying attention to the quality of the movement. The quality of the return. Can you smooth things out? Do both legs feel the same or is one side a little different, is one side more hesitant than the other? Does one have better range or less range?

Paws once again.

These simple moves for the central and lower body takes the key movement just one step further.

Now you're going to shift to your upper body.

Position: Knees bent. Arms comfortably at or near your sides.

Movement: As if you are going to do a snow angel.

Do: Slide both arms away from your sides. If it is comfortable for you to slide them up to shoulder height then please slide your arms to a comfortable position as if you're making a snow angel or jumping jack.

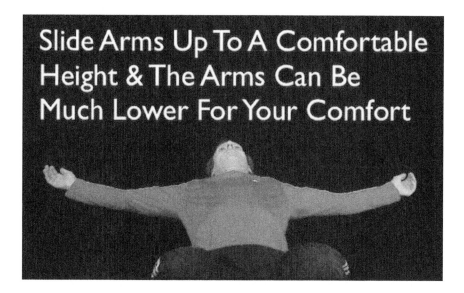

Rest or pause in the comfortable position with the arms away from the side.

Undo: Slowly allow the arms to come back down to where they can rest near or away from your side comfortably.

Do: Easily slide the arms out and away from your sides.

Feeling: Can you feel your shoulders contracting? Do you feel certain muscles in your neck contract as your arms slide up a little higher?

Undo: Slowly release.

Feeling: Notice how well you can release. Make sure you are releasing slowly and not in a hurry to go back so quickly. Can you feel your shoulders readjusting?

Paws.

Do: Slide your arms up to make a snow angel.

Undo: Slide your arms back down.

Feeling: Were you conscious of your breathing or were you breath holding during the movement?

The more you are able to breathe and move, it's more likely the movement will be easier to follow along.

Repeat the movement and check in with your breathing as you are moving.

If you catch yourself breath holding, notice what happens as you hold your breath. Is the movement easier or more difficult?

Position: Now slide your arms up to shoulder height if it is comfortable otherwise to your comfortable position. Then bend your arms so the wrist lie in the air above the bent elbow. Your palms can face forwards or towards your feet. This will be the starting position.

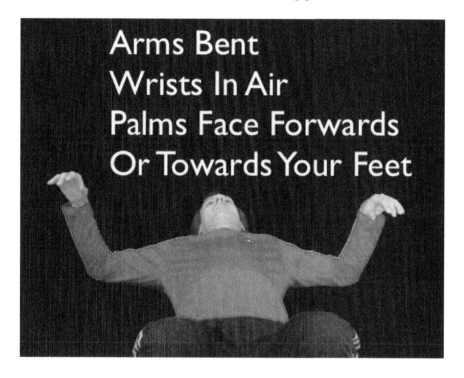

A key is to do the movement gently without a lot of force.

This is about the quality and the feel of a movement and its release.

Do: Breathe in and attempt to slide the slide the shoulder blades in towards each other.

Undo: Slowly allow for the release.

Sensing: Notice how well your shoulders release. How well do they let go when you do it slowly.

Paws.

Do: Breathe in and bring the shoulders back.

Feeling: Do you get the sense your chest is coming forwards?

Undo: Slowly allow for the release.

Sensing: Notice if your chest falls back slightly.

Some of these self-observations are very, very subtle when you work in this slow micro-movement environment.

One more time.

Do: Slide the shoulder blades back in towards each other.

Undo: Release slowly.

Feeling: Can you allow for the release to be smooth and in your control?

Then turn off those efforts and allow your arms to slide back down towards the neutral position resting comfortably at or near your sides without any residual tension. You can rest with your knees bent or legs extended.

Feeling: Tune into the feelings and sensations you are aware of in this moment in your shoulder area, in your chest, and in your neck.

Putting It All Together

Position: Now let's put this pattern together with your arms at or near your sides. Your knees are bent, feet flat.

Do: As you breathe in, allow the knees to drift apart as you make the snow angel with your arms.

This time as your arms travel out into the snow angel position, you can allow them to remain lengthened.

Do: Slide the shoulder blades back in towards each other.

Undo: Allow the shoulders to release and come to a rest in this position.

Undo: Simultaneously, bring both the arms and knees in.

Feeling: Can you time the return to be equal so all four limbs come to a resting position at the same time?

Remember to un-do slowly. If one limb gets ahead of another, it is OK.

Paws.

Movement: Repeat again.

Do: Allow the knees to drift apart as the arms drift out into the snow angel position. Then once you're in the snow angel position as the knees are out, slide the shoulder blades in towards each other.

Undo: Allow that to release as you breath accordingly.

If the return can be one long exhalation or if you need a series of in and out breaths by all means do so.

Then come to a paws.

Movement: In the third and final attempt.

Do: Allow the knees to drift apart as well as the arms drifting apart. As you slide the shoulder blades in, attempt to move the knees towards the surface so you can...

Feeling: Feel what happens in your back as you take the knees out and the shoulders in.

Undo: Slowly allow for those muscles to release.

Undo: Then begin to time the movement of the arms and legs to where they started from.

Then come back to paws.

Final Move

One final movement to tie all the pieces together.

Do: Draw the knees in as you bring the arms into your sides and gently lift your head forwards as if you're going to look at your knees. (This doesn't have to be a big lift).

Feeling: Notice the feeling or the contractions you are doing in the front part of your body, from your neck, your chest, your abdomen, your inner legs, the sides where your arms are coming in.

Undo: Slowly release and allow your body to come back, your head, your upper back comes back to the surface. Your arms slide away from the side going back to neutral or a more comfortable position as the legs move back to neutral too.

Now you've created the ability to flex the back since you took the tension out of the backwards pull and normal contraction which happens as a normal "on" signal of the go-getter.

Paws with your knees bent or your legs extended.

Feeling: Notice whatever feelings or sense perceptions arise in this moment. Feel your contact with the surface. Is it the same or a little different compared to when you first began or checked in.

After some 30 seconds or a minute or as long as you need to be sufficient to feel yourself and any feelings or sensations which arise...

Now you're ready to go-go-go again and be as quick as a cheetah.

To calm down those amped up feelings and sensations of a tight, stiff, tensed back is what you actively engaged in. Then you followed up with a movement to feel the now more lengthened muscles in the back.

Recap

You still followed the same 3 step method that you learned in chapter 4.

You were doing a movement more geared towards your posture, circumstances or on those days when you're feeling amped up.

You did a particular movement sequence from one part of the key movement from chapter 5 as well as the parts to the final global movement pattern we did in the last 2 movements.

All of this can be done in a matter of minutes when you wake-up in the morning. This is the same kind of thing you can do in the late afternoon or in the evening before you go to sleep to take out any accumulated stress or tension from the day.

Then you're set up to go-go-go the very next morning albeit from a more relaxed and responsive body. You can prepare yourself to handle all the stresses and tensions that arise.

To use all the simple tools of mindful movement, breathing and conscious awareness to restore and re-energize your system shifting from the "on" button to the "off" button. Your muscles will remember to stay relaxed for more longer periods of time.

In the next chapter, we're going to look at what happens as a result of when things go oops or we take on falls, traumas and accidents which keeps our muscles at bay.

Turn the page now to learn a set of movements for when people, places and things bump into us or we bump into them.

Chapter 8

What can I do for Oops, Falls, Strains, Accidents and Trauma?

Oops, you bumped into something or something bumped you off track. Do you know the struggles of limping around? Has the bracing, stiff, cuffs-like hold let go? Are you still hobbling in spite of your best efforts? Are those niggling injuries beginning to add up and you can't shake them off like you used to? Were you told you had to have crutches on the way back to getting your giddyup back?

Did they tell you one leg is shorter than the other? Did they say you are or do you feel short waisted?

If you've fallen, taken a big hit or suffered from trauma. Any move in any direction can cause you to wince, guard and hold yourself together. Avoiding that certain discomfort or pain, we guard ourself with our super protector powers.

If left "on" for too long a time, we somehow manage to limp, hobble or throw our hips around as well as we can though in our hearts we know how we used to move more easily.

A Squirrels Story on the Power of Pandiculation

One day I saw a squirrel fall out of a tree, landing right on its head. Systematically, it was able to put itself back together and triumphantly walk back into the woods.

Mesmerized by the squirrel's circumstances, I wondered how do animals help themselves when it comes to injury, falls and accidents.

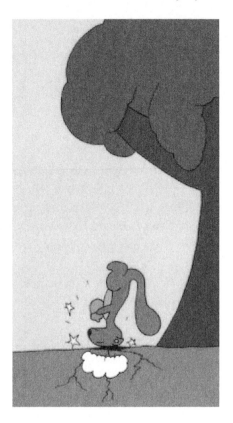

What I saw is the very same method they use to keep developing their foundation for movement.

Naturally, they "go to" what they know. They go back into creating a smaller space in order to allow for the larger space to let go or restore itself.

When we experienced ankle sprains or strains as a child at some point we recovered. When we fall, how do we brace ourselves up today? Do we ice it, stay off of it, get some type of brace or get some crutches as we wince around for a length of time?

Simply through the act of a pandiculation we can lose our crutches, binds and tension patterns which defy letting go with other methods.

Losing Crutches

A woman came to me with crutches. She wanted to get back to her Bollywood dancing. In less than an hour, she was able to do some movements which freed her up.

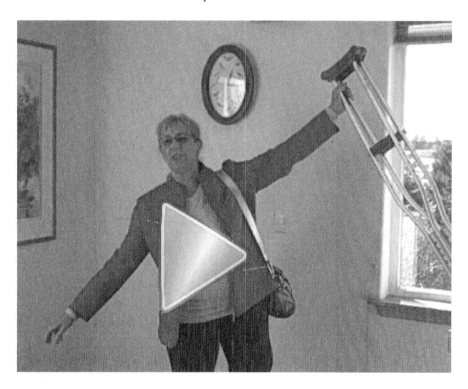

Watch this video at http://youtu.be/3KIGG128fFY. Watch and listen to her story.

When we suffer a fall or an accident, our body tends to go back into a protective holding pattern. The natural thing to do is to protect ourself from further hurt or discomfort.

Accumulating Trauma

In the game of soccer I enjoy, I get knocked to the ground, collide and go bump quite often. Each one of these moments is in some way a mini-trauma as the muscles will re-contract to protect. If I don't do anything afterwards, or ASAP, the contraction patterns begin to lock-down and hold us in check.

The binding process starts. As we age, the stiffness, the binds and high tension patterns may have been or begun as a result of some type of trauma to our body.

We can accumulate these patterns which can be layered over other traumas. We can think of this as a temporary ongoing phenomena since the signals to hold on, keep doing their job according to the set program for many, many, many years in some cases.

Letting Go

When we go back in this mindful, conscientious way of moving ourself about, the brain will begin to free up the tissues back to the comfort zone.

In some physical therapy traditions, you may have heard you need to break up the scar tissue. That mass of tissue which can feel jumbled, mangled together, or feels like a thick glue when you move around.

In our animal approach, we're going to move with what your nervous system is presenting. We go "with" in order to unlock.

Shift in Posture

Say we're hobbling or we're moving, tilting, or bracing away from the side of discomfort. Our postures tend to shift off to one side or the other. We may bear our weight then more on one leg to ease things.

Maybe Mom was carrying one of our siblings on her one hip. We watched her do it this way and adopted the very same posture. We began to stand more on one leg than the other. It's possible the waist on the side began to tighten, become shorter as the hip on that side tends to rise when we shift and bear weight and hold ourself in this manner.

This kind of adaptation just sneaks up on us and before we know it, the pattern has been reinforced and is ours to keep for as long as we show it.

A Stitch in our Side

Our short waisted-ness may have begun so simply and innocently. Then as we began to run and we'd get a certain stitch in our side. Our muscles would cramp or take some of the air out of us. Maybe we didn't know how to relieve it or somehow it would resolve itself on its own.

You're going to learn some simple movements which will help release the on-going phenomena of holding patterns, stitches, and postures where we either bear our weight to one side more than the other. Similar to a driver who leans on the armrest shifting their upper body one way as the lower body is the other as the car travels down the road.

To begin the process of freeing up a limp, a fall, a past strain. Once again, we'll work near the center of gravity to change things from the inside out.

Movement Pattern To Help Release Trauma

The movement pattern will be broken down into parts and then put together at the end.

Remember, your comfort is important. You may need to use a pillow, towel or other cushy things to support yourself.

Again, the 3 step method you learned in chapter 4 is key to pandiculating tension and restoring muscular function.

Since many of us are combinations of adapted postures, you can move with your present set of circumstances. All it takes is a micro-move, a small self-corrective movement or using your imagination to use the 3 step method.

Position: Lie on the side you are presently more comfortable on. The side which is up in the air or further from the ground, will be the first side to be addressed.

Lower Body Position: On your side, knees bent, one leg atop another. As if you're a chair seated sideways.

Keep the ankles underneath your knees. Ideally your ankles can rest slightly in front or directly underneath rather than slightly behind or more bent backwards.

Upper Body Position: The ideal position is for the arm to act as a pillow for the head. The arm can be straightened above your head. Some of you will choose to keep it bent. If you need a pillow for support, use it.

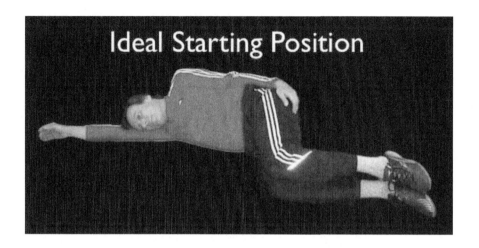

Ideal Starting Position

To modify this in case there is too much upper body tension where the upper body is being pulled forwards slightly. It is OK initially to lie a bit curled forward since this is your present comfort zone.

As things begin to free up with the upper body from doing the 2nd part of the key movement or the withdrawal movement from chapter 6, the upper body will feel freer to open and be in the more ideal position.

Ideal Overall Position: a straight line from the hips up to the shoulder and head with the arm straight. The bent knees can be out in front of you, slightly higher or lower depending once again on your comfort zone.

In the same way we developed ourself in the first place with same-sided and contralateral movements, we unbind ourself from trauma with certain patterns followed by other ones to keep freeing ourself and improving our overall movement ability and capacity.

When it comes to recovering from trauma, you want to move gently, easily and lightly even to the point of imagining the movements if the situation calls for it, especially when we're in those wincing, bracing states.

There may be moments when say your ribs are hurting so much that any movement or the best medicine itself, laughter can set off a painful response. Laughing and in being in pain is just part of life's circumstances.

Be mindful, careful and again incorporate breathing with movement.

Lower Body Movement

Focus your attention on your lower body. You'll begin with your hip.

Do: As if you could slide the hip up towards your armpit, begin to slide the hip upwards in the direction of the under arm or armpit.

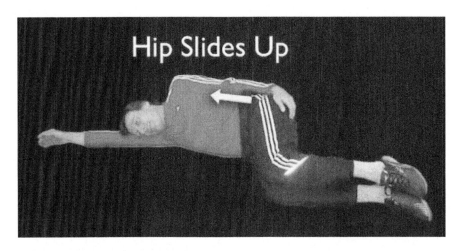

Undo: Slowly release the hip.

Paws.

Repeat. Do: As you slide the hip up...

Feeling: Notice what or where it is you are contracting or tensing.

Undo: Release the contraction or tension slowly.

Feeling: Do you get a sense the muscles along your side or waist area are beginning to let go?

You may or may not notice if any of the muscles are letting go.

Paws.

Place your hand on or at your waist level.

Do: Gently slide the hip up again.

Feeling: Notice if there is any sensation, movement, contraction or tension building underneath your finger or thumb.

Undo: Allow for the release to occur.

Paws. Take your hand away and tune into that part of yourself as you...

Do: Slide the hip up

.

Feeling: Feel the muscles contracting or tensing where you previously had your hand, in your waist.

Undo: Allow for the slow release.

Feeling: How well, how smooth are you able to let go as the hip rolls back down to the place where it started?

Paws.

Tune into the feelings and sensations around your waist area.

Notice how you are breathing.

Upper Body Movement

Now focus on your upper body. Have your arm rest along your side.

Focus on your armpit.

Do: Begin to pull your armpit down towards the hip.

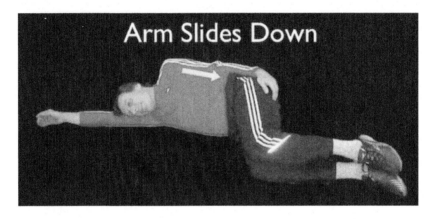

Undo: Allow the contracted, tensed area to slowly release back up to where you started.

Paws.

Do: Contract the armpit downwards.

Feeling: Feel the shoulder moving down towards the hip.

Undo: Release slowly.

Feeling: What or where do you feel letting go underneath your armpit, in your ribcage and in your shoulder?

Paws.

Repeat the movement again gently and easily.

Do: Slide the shoulder down towards the hip.

Undo: Allow for the slow release.

Feeling: How well, how smooth, how easily and effortless can you allow for the release of that contraction or tension you generated in the movement?

Paws.

Feeling: Tune into the feelings and sensations around your ribs, and underneath your armpit. Notice how you are breathing.

Upper and Lower Body Movement

Let's put those two parts of the movement together.

Do: Breathe out as you slide the hip up and the shoulder down towards the hip.

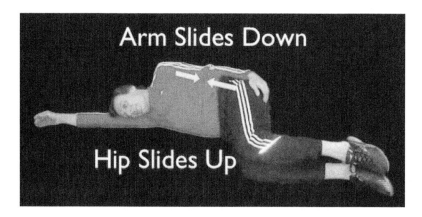

Feeling: Feel how your side tightens and tenses in this movement.

Undo: Allow the muscles of your side to slowly release as the air comes back into you.

Paws. Turn everything off and come to a rest.

When you're ready. Repeat by exhaling...

Do: Slide the hip up as the shoulder moves down.

Feeling: Notice how the entire side begins to tighten and contract as you are moving.

Undo: Slowly ease the tension off.

Feeling: How well does the shoulder slide away from the hip? How well does the hip move away from the shoulder?

Paws. Let your breathe regulate.

When your breath is easy and comfortable, once again...

Do: Slide your hip up towards your shoulder, as your shoulder moves down towards the hip.

Undo: Ease off of the contraction and tension you've created.

Feeling: Notice how well and smooth you can allow the hip and shoulder to move back towards their relative starting points. How do you feel your ribcage participating?

Paws.

Now you'll take this one step further.

Do: Gently move the arm out in front of you. Hand on the surface. Begin to slide it upwards towards your other hand on the floor. At the same time, slide your upper leg downwards so a straight line is formed as you gently reach both the arm and leg.

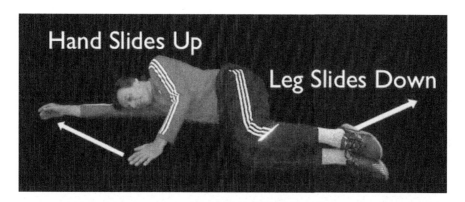

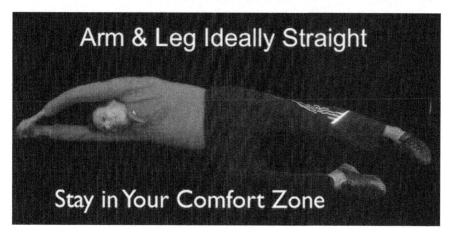

Undo: Allow yourself to release back to where it started with the leg bent and hand out in front of you.

Paws.

Do: Slide the hip up as you bring the shoulder down.

Undo: Allow for the release.

Paws.

Do: Move the arm slowly away from your side and as you begin to straighten the arm, do so with the leg.

Feeling: What is happening as you straighten both the arm and leg? Can you sense your other side now contracting or lifting up off of the ground?

Undo: As you release...

Feeling: Does your side closest to the ground begin to let go?

Gently and easily allow your limbs to come back to where you started. Turn everything off and come to a rest.

One more time.

Do: Hip up, shoulder down.

Undo: Slowly release yourself.

Feeling: Pay attention to the quality of your release.

After the release and momentary paws...

Do: Slide the arm out in front of you. As the arm begins to extend, extend the leg downwards.

Feeling: Feel what is happening in the side on the surface.

Undo: Allow for the release.

Feeling: Sense what happens to the muscles in your side nearest the surface.

Slowly bring the arm and leg back to where you started.

Paws. Turn off all of your efforts and rest while lying on your side.

Tune into any feelings or sense perceptions you're aware of in this moment.

After some sufficient time to tune in, roll onto your back.

Rest with either your knees bent or legs extended.

As you lie there, compare from the inside. Feel what your waist feels like. Feel what your ribs feel like. Feel what your hip feels like.

Compare those feelings and sensations with your other side waist, your other side ribs, your other side hip.

Do you feel different on one side compared to the other?

If so, what's the difference feel like to you?

Continue to lie there for as long as you'd like.

Change Sides

Now begin to reposition yourself to the other side so you are lying in that similar position of the chair seated sideways with your legs together and straight arm (if it's possible) underneath your head to act as a pillow.

Focus your attention to the hip closest to the ceiling.

Do: Slide the hip up towards your armpit.

Undo: Slowly allow that hip to release.

Paws.

Do: Slide the hip up.

Feeling: Sense what it is you are contracting.

Undo: Slowly allow the hip to slide back down.

Feeling: How does this side compares to the other side?

Paws.

Do: Slide the hip and contract the muscles on your side.

Feeling: Do you get a sense that the other hip is sliding downwards in relationship to this hip sliding upwards?

Undo: Begin to release the contraction of your side. Allow the hip to roll back to where it started.

Paws your efforts.

As you rest, tune into the feelings and sensations on this side.

Now focus your attention on your shoulder and armpit area.

Do: Begin to bring down the shoulder as if you could bring your armpit down towards the hip.

Undo: Undo the movement with a slow, easy, and gradual release.

Paws.

Then repeat, easily and gently.

Do: Pull the shoulder down towards the hip.

Feeling: Feel the area you are tensing or contracting as you move.

Undo: As smoothly as you can, allow for a smooth release.

Feeling: Is your release ratchety? If it is, slow down your release even more.

Paws.

Do: On your third and final attempt, allow for this movement to be the easiest and lightest effort while tuning into what and where is tensing, pulling, contracting or moving.

Feeling: How does your opposite side shoulder move?

Undo: Twice as slow as you did the last time, allow for a very slow and controlled release.

Paws.

Tune into the feelings and sensations created. Notice the feelings in your armpit, in your ribs.

Notice how you are breathing.

Upper and Lower Body Movement

Do: As the hip slides up, bring the shoulder down as if they could meet.

Undo: Allow for the hip to move away from the shoulder as the shoulder moves away from the hip.

Paws.

Repeat. Do: Shoulder down, hip up.

Feeling: As this side begins to get shorter, does the side on the ground allow for a lengthening?

Undo: Undo the movement.

Feeling: How well does your side, do your ribs, underneath your armpit... how well does all of this let go? How easy is it for the hip and shoulder to slide back to where they started from?

Paws.

On your third and final attempt. Move easily, lightly.

Do: Slide the hip up as the shoulder moves down.

Feeling: Where are the efforts taking place?

Undo: Ease those efforts off.

Feeling: Notice how your hips are responding? How are your shoulders responding... how is your waist responding? How does your ribcage move?

Paws.

Do: Then allow for the arm closest to the ceiling to begin to move out in front of you to straighten the arm above your head as you straighten the leg downwards.

Feeling: Feel how the waist on the surface begins to contract to allow for the arm and leg to comfortably lengthen without any strain.

Undo: Take your time as you release the waist nearer the ground, begin to bend the leg and arm and bring your limbs back to where you started from.

Paws. Tune into how your are breathing in this moment.

Do: Hip up, shoulder down.

Undo: Allow for the release.

Paws.

Do: Bring the arm out in front of you, begin to lengthen the arm and leg at the same time.

Feeling: Sense how the waist begins to open as the waist nearer the ground begins to contract and lifts up so there is no strain in the arm or in the leg.

Undo: Release the waist while at the same time begin to bring the arm and the leg back down to where it started.

Once you're there, turn off all of your efforts and Paws.

Do: One final time, easily, lightly bring the hip up and the shoulder down.

Undo: Allow for that release to occur.

Paws.

Do: Then begin to bring the arm out in front of you. Slide it upwards as the leg moves downwards. Allow for the side along the surface to play its part.

Undo: Ease off all of your efforts until you come in for a complete rest.

As you lie and rest on your side, tune into how well you are breathing.

What other feelings or sense perceptions are you aware of in this moment?

After your rest, gently and easily roll yourself onto your back and rest again with either your legs extended or knees bent, whichever is more comfortable for you.

Feeling: Notice how the side you just worked with feels. Feel the waist. Feel the ribs. Feel the hip. Feel the entire side.

Is it different? Has it changed from only a few moments ago?

After a sufficient rest, that's the end of this particular movement pattern.

Restoration

When we've had falls or trauma and we tend to hobble, favor or limp, you now have a direct pattern that you can begin to play with. Either through the actual movement itself or in those bracing, wincing moments, you can merely imagine yourself doing the movements.

Within about 72 hours, you'll begin to notice, if not sooner, how things will begin to move more freely. Even if you just do these in your minds eye or imagination.

This simple movement pattern can begin the process of restoring yourself back from being tilted over to one side, after a collision or fall. This can help us out of the habit of leaning or bearing weight primarily on one side.

When you're upright, you may begin to sense if you are indeed bearing your weight more on one side than the other. You may begin to sense the contractions in your side, waist or ribs.

After the Movement

Stand up after doing a pattern such as this one. When you stand, imagine you are lying on your back. Take some time and notice how you are standing as a result of doing this particular movement pattern. How do you bear your weight?

Is it more even or do you list or favor one side over the other?

After you stand, take a small walk. How does your walk feel to you? Can you feel your shoulders moving? How do your hips move? How do feel your ribs participating?

Walking Game

Here's a game to try. Keep one hip up and the shoulder down as you walk in this manner as if you're titled to the side.

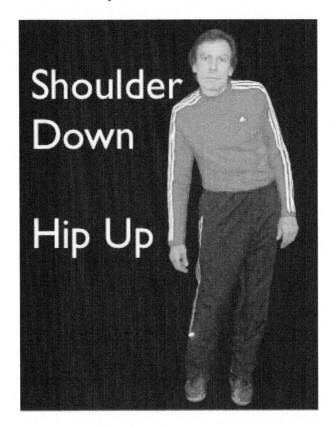

You're consciously hobbling on that side. Notice what this bend feels like to you. Take several steps and then release that side. Play the game on the other side to tilt over and feel how your walking changes. Then allow for the release.

As you keep walking, feel the movement and the actions in your sides. Your sides may have become a forgotten area. Once we've been traumatized, have enough accidents or falls, we shield away from a particular side... the brain begins to check out and our parts get carried along by other parts of our self.

The muscles forget to move and other parts are called into action to hobble, even to the point of getting used to it and accustoming ourself in being. For some of us, this can last for any length of period.

With sufficient trauma, we may need to move around the trauma so the entire system can begin to be free again.

Recap

Work with your more affected side to begin with.

Do the simple movement pattern for both the upper and lower body. Then do the combination movement. Tune in and repeat on the other side. Then stand up to notice how you are standing. Then feel free to play the walking game.

In the series of Move Like an Animal books to follow, we'll take this particular movement pattern and begin to expand this out and add more layers. This will give you a good starting point which you can combine with the key movement pattern.

In the next chapter, you'll get a plan & final thoughts to put all the movement patterns in this book together so you can freely *move like an animal* again and again.

Last Thoughts

How to Put it All Together and Move Like an Animal for a Comfortable Life

To move like an animal and recapture our childlike feelings of freedom is easy, since it is our natural birthright to move well.

You simply rekindle the natural act of pandiculation. This re-establishes our foundation for more comfortable movement.

R-O-A-R Your Way Back

To Recover-Over-Any-Restriction (R-O-A-R) simply pandiculate with the 3 step method.

Unwinding from our postural or movement difficulties, stiffness, high tension levels, stress and niggling injuries is easily afforded by the system of somatics exercises which uses pandiculation at its heart.

By recognizing how the brain is set up to serve us, we can wield its powers to remain comfortable for life.

How to Best Use the Movements

Just as any healthy vertebrate animal begins the day, you too can pandiculate out the tightness and stiffness which occurs at night. This resetting process takes a few minutes and you can begin the day with the simple key movement you learned in chapter 5.

Anytime you feel it is necessary to reset your body, by all means do so. Remember, healthy animals reset 40 - 50 times per day. It's no wonder they move so incredibly well.

At night, before you retire, you may want to take out some of the stress and tension which builds up during the course of a busy, hectic day. Watch Fido, right before he retires, he'll do the same. Good night; sleep well.

Plan A

You can systematically work your way through chapters 5 - 8, or, after you learn the key movement, begin with which movements serve you the best.

Ideally, you repeat the movement sequence in each chapter for a week to 10 days, then move on to the next one. This will give you something to practice for either 28 days or 40, depending on how much time you want to explore.

Notice any changes each day in your ability to both do and feel or sense the movements. Also notice whether things begin to loosen up overall as you progress.

Plan B

Alternatively, you can begin with chapter 5. Then either pick the next appropriate chapter or follow this series—chapter 5 the first day, chapter 7 the second day, chapter 6 the third day, chapter 8 the fourth day and then complete with chapter 5 on the fifth day. Then rinse and repeat until you've come full circle 7 to 10 more times.

Plan C

Take an afternoon off. Explore all the somatics exercises and movement routines as if you're attending a workshop. You can rotate through all the movements taking breaks in between each movement series.

Listen Up

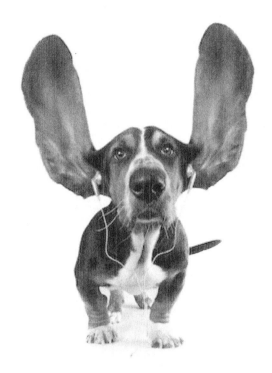

To get to the true spirit in how to do these movements, you can listen to the series of audio recordings which will give you the pace and timing. If you purchased this book, you can access the audio recordings by contacting us at support@gravitywerks.com.

Sensory and Movement Skills Development

When it comes to our sensory development, this may take some time to redevelop. No worries. First you have to learn what the movement is, then attempt or imagine the movement. Your movement skills and understanding will improve with practice.

Later on, the sensitivity and control re-establish themselves. As you refine this with practice, you delve deeper into the feelings and sense perceptions which arise as a result of conscious movement.

All movement can produce feelings when we choose to tap into this reservoir of sentience. Our great actors have known how to wield this with the way they carry their postures so we can believe the characters they portray. When we fully feel our feelings and couple that with our movements, then our believe-ability and credibility arises too.

We can see and feel our moments of achievement, glory and joy as well as the other side of loss, despair and grief. We can all move through life's ever changing set of circumstances more freely. To go with the flow and be more comfortable throughout one's life can be afforded when we consciously play with our movement abilities. Our sensitivity to our own plight and that of others can be enhanced—and we can help each other move onwards.

The Key of Differentiation

To give you a heads up on what's to come... Differentiation is the key to ongoing vitality. Both the brain and body thrive when novelty is introduced.

Since we have 17 layers of muscles to organize, along with our 600 muscles to regain function, we have many sensitive receptor sites. In fact, there are far more in the fascia which covers our muscles, joints and tendons.

With all of our layers and sense receptors, there is plenty we can do to artfully articulate and get ourselves out of our own tricky and sticky sets of circumstances.

Coming Soon

In the future book series, you'll learn how to handle neck pain, lower back pain, troublesome hands, stiff and ailing knees, bothersome hips, sore shoulders and more. We'll even delve into things you can do for yourself when you experience tight jaws, and aching feet too.

If you've got pain or discomfort, we'll figure out a way to consciously move you back to comfort with simple pandiculations, via the system of somatics exercises, to reset the body.

In the meantime, you can check out the additional free training I have to offer at GravityWerks.com.

Be Comfortable, Move Well... Move Like An Animal!

Edward Barrera

Hanna Somatic Educator®, H.S.E.
Holistic Health Advisor, H.H.A.
Founder of Gravity Werks

Epilogue

This book is dedicated to my former training partner and favorite pandiculator, Buddy.

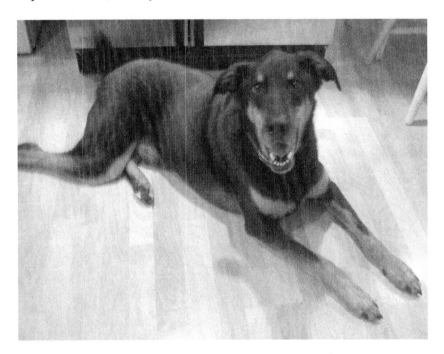

His boundless love and his art of pandiculation was a simple daily act. In his last two years, he lived with Addison's disease. I was truly blessed to be in his company during the best of times and his trying times. In the last moment of his life, while he continued to strive to live, he gave one final pandiculation and comfortably relaxed his way into the hereafter.

He showed those around him; more than to Move Like an Animal.

References

Doidge, Norman, The Brain That Changes Itself: Stories of Personal Triumph from the Frontiers of Brain Science, 2007.

Hanna, Thomas, Somatics: Reawakening The Mind's Control Of Movement, Flexibility, And Health, 1988.

Heller, Joseh & Henkin, William A., Bodywise: An Introduction to Hellerwork for Regaining Flexibility and Well-Being, North Atlantic Books, 2004.

Keleman, Stanley, Emotional Anatomy, Center Press, 1989.

Juhan, Deane, Job's Body, A Handbook for Bodywork, Barrytown/ Station Hill Press, 2003.

Myers, Thomas, Anatomy Trains: Myofascial Meridians for Manual and Movement Therapists, Churchill Livingstone, 2008.

Sharkey, John, The Concise Book of Neuromuscular Therapy: A Trigger Point Manual, Lotus Publishing, 2008.

Siff, Mel C., Facts and Fallacies of Fitness, Perform Better, 2003.

Walusinski, O., The Mystery of Yawning in Physiology and Disease, (Frontiers of Neurology and Neuroscience). S. Karger, 2010.

Printed in Great Britain
by Amazon